A GUIDE TO LIVING WITH LUPUS
FOR YOU AND YOUR FAMILY

Coping
with
Lupus

ROBERT H. PHILLIPS, Ph.D.

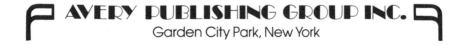
AVERY PUBLISHING GROUP INC.
Garden City Park, New York

The medical information and procedures contained in this book are not intended as a substitute for consulting your physician. All matters regarding your physical health should be supervised by a medical professional.

In-house editor: Cynthia J. Eriksen
Typesetters: Straight Creek Company, Denver, Colorado

Library of Congress Cataloging-in-Publication Data

Phillips, Robert H., 1948–
    Coping with lupus : a guide to living with lupus for you and your family / Robert H. Phillips.
        p.   cm.
    Includes bibliographical references and index.
    ISBN 0-89529-475-3
    1. Systemic lupus erythematosus—Psychological aspects.
    2. Systemic lupus erythematosus—Patients—Family relationships.
    3. Adjustment (Psychology)   I. Title.
RC924.5.L85P45   1991
616.97—dc20   90-1270
                                                        CIP

Printed in the United States of America

10 9 8 7 6 5 4 3 2

Contents

Dedication

This book is lovingly dedicated to my wife, Sharon, and my three sons, Michael, Larry, and Steven; my parents, sister, and grandparents; all my other relatives and in-laws; and my friends.

This book is also dedicated to the memories of Murray and Doris Shaer—Murray, a wonderful, inspiring man who dedicated a significant portion of his life to helping those with lupus, and Doris, one of the most incredibly good-natured, giving, and compassionate people I've ever known, and one of the guiding forces behind the development of the Lupus Foundation of America.

Finally, this book is adoringly dedicated to the memory of my grandfather, Mickey Kurzrock—a man who was so well-loved, and who, through his joie de vivre, constantly demonstrated the advantages of coping with illness. Thank you, Skipper.

Acknowledgments

Appreciative words of thanks must be accorded some very special people who provided invaluable assistance in the preparation of this book. Thanks to Paula Goldstein, Brenda McCormack, and Carol Goldklang for their critical review, helpful suggestions, and belief in this project. Thanks to Robert Marcus, M.D., for his informative review of the manuscript. Thanks to Shelley Markowitz and Sharon Balaban for the hours spent transcribing, revising, and typing the manuscript. Thanks to the thousands of members of the Lupus Foundation of America who provided such important insight into the critical aspects of living with lupus. Finally, thanks to Ron Carr, M.D., Ph.D., for professional evaluation of the highest caliber—his expertise, guidance, and friendship are highly valued.

Preface

The diagnosis of systemic lupus erythematosus can have a major impact on you and your family. No kidding! Many questions will come to mind. Some of them can be answered by physicians or other professionals. Others may be answered by the relatively few books or articles on the subject. However, many questions cannot be answered. Why? Scientists just don't know the answers. This can be upsetting. Also upsetting is the feeling of isolation you may experience, the feeling that you're alone because no one understands. Knowing that you have a chronic illness can be depressing.

Medical science has been making progress in controlling lupus. There is every chance that this will enable you to lead a longer, more normal and productive life. But what about the psychological effects of lupus? A major factor determining your potential to lead a normal, emotionally stable life is how well you cope with the strain of having a chronic illness such as lupus.

Heavy stuff? You bet it is! But it shows why this book was written in the first place. This book, chock-full of information, suggestions, and techniques, was written to help you, the members of you family, and your friends learn how to cope with lupus.

The first part of the book presents basic information about lupus: what it is, what the symptoms are, how to treat it, and so on. The other sections deal with different aspects of living with the disease, including how to cope with your emotions, changes in lifestyle, and living with others. These are all important aspects of coping with this or any other chronic condition. We will explore them in detail, and you'll find suggestions and strategies as well as illustrative examples for each component. In fact, a lot of the information you'll read can (and does!) apply to any chronic condition. In this book, however, the main focus is on your life with lupus.

Although you will read about many of the symptoms of lupus, you must remember that no one with this illness ever has *all* of the symptoms. Symptoms occur differently in each individual. Similarly, the psychological effects of having lupus also vary with each person who is diagnosed with the illness. You are a unique person. However, after reading the book, you'll realize that you're not alone; others share what you feel. This can be reassuring. Even though a lot of similarities may exist between you and others with lupus, your own life with lupus—the way it affects you and the way you experience it—will not be exactly the same as anyone else's. Therefore, it will be up to *you* to use the suggestions and strategies in the book to help you cope as well as you possibly can.

Researchers are working hard, trying to find a cure for lupus. But until that time, you'll have to live with it. I hope this book is of help to you and your family. Remember: You can *always* improve the quality of your life.

Robert H. Phillips, Ph.D.
Center for Coping with Chronic Conditions
Long Island, NY

Foreword

Systemic lupus erythematosus (SLE), more loosely known as lupus, is a chronic disease involving the body's immune system. Individuals who are afflicted with this illness can suffer a myriad of varying manifestations that can affect almost any part of the body. The manifestation can be quite minimal or extremely severe and even life threatening, and they can appear and disappear with frustrating unpredictability, lasting anywhere from a few days to several months or more. Thus, those with this illness frequently can go for months or even years while physicians vainly try to make the diagnosis, and it is not uncommon, especially in the milder cases, for such patients to be labelled as neurotics or chronic complainers. Even after the diagnosis is made and the appropriate therapy is instituted, the patient has to live with the knowledge that the illness is not yet curable, and even though treatment has improved dramatically over the last decade, it is still far from ideal since the drugs used in many cases have significant untoward side effects. Obviously, all of this creates a life situation in which significant psychological stress is a constant companion of the patient, not only in terms of the disease per se, but also because in the face of all of the above, the individual must still interact with family, friends, employers, and strangers as we all do. It doesn't take much of an imagination to understand that lupus patients have to cope not only with internal stresses, but also with the responses of the people around them, responses which at times can be as infuriating and frustrating as the disease itself.

Although a number of books have been written on lupus, both highly technical for physicians and in lay language for the general public, there has been a crying need for a comprehensive source book for patients and their families on how to cope with the psychological problems that such an illness produces. Bob Phillips is eminently qualified to have written such a book. He is a practicing psychologist who counsels many lupus patients because he has developed a special interest in the problems of this disease. He is also on the medical council of the Lupus Foundation of America, and has served as a member of the National Board of Directors of the Lupus Foundation. He has written this book with understanding and compassion, and has included not only a comprehensive discussion of the kinds of reactions patients must deal with, but also many practical suggestions to help them do so. Having read the manuscript, I would like to say that I only wish all lupus patients could be so lucky as to have access to someone like Dr. Phillips, and that by writing this book, he has given them, in some sense at least, that access.

Ronald I. Carr, M.D., Ph.D.
Associate Professor of Medicine
Associate Professor of Microbiology
Dalhousie University Faculty of Medicine
Halifax, Nova Scotia, Canada

PART I
Lupus—An Overview

1

What Is Lupus?

Susan, a 29-year-old mother of one, had not been feeling well. She had been feeling very tired for a long time, and was experiencing more and more pain in many joints of her body. Seeing a number of different doctors had resulted in several different diagnoses, but no treatment was helping her to feel better. Finally, she went to yet another physician who gave her a complete physical, including all kinds of blood tests. After extensive analysis of the tests performed, he was now meeting with Susan in his consultation room to explain the findings. Susan nervously approached the chair by his desk and sat down. Her husband of six years sat by her side. The doctor looked at her and wasted no time in telling her, "Susan, you have lupus." Susan's immediate reaction was very similar to the immediate reaction of many individuals diagnosed as having lupus. Trembling, she looked at the doctor and exclaimed, "What's lupus?"

So, what is lupus? Lupus is the more commonly known name for systemic lupus erythematosus. But what is it? Lupus falls into the category of diseases known as autoimmune diseases. To understand why, and to understand what happens in lupus, it is important to be aware of how our immune system operates.

WHAT DO OUR ANTIBODIES DO?

The immune system is a very important part of our bodies. This system is essential in protecting us from infection, in addition to helping to maintain normal body functioning.

Imagine our immune system as a fort in a city. Inside the fort there are thousands and thousands of soldiers who sit in readiness, waiting to go outside the fort and go to different areas in the city to fight evil and destroy the enemy. Normally, the immune system (the fort) produces antibodies (the soldiers) and cells (the tanks) that fight foreign substances (the enemies), such as bacteria, viruses, and other germs, throughout the body (the city). In lupus there seems to be a malfunction in some of the cells of the immune system. For some reason that is not completely understood, there are soldiers inside the fort who try to destroy the city and perhaps the fort itself. This is what characterizes lupus. In lupus, normal, healthy tissue in the body is attacked by the increased amount of antibodies (the deranged soldiers). This attack leads to a kind of allergic reaction. You may be able to see evidence of inflammation in certain parts of the body where the attack is taking place. This is why lupus is also considered to be an inflammatory disease. The inflamed areas are usually reddish in color, tender to the touch, and often painful. Since individuals with lupus have such high amounts of self-fighting antibodies, lupus is called an autoimmune disease. This means that for some reason, you have in a sense become allergic to parts of your own body, although it is not the same kind of allergy that you might experience if you had hay fever or another common allergy.

WHERE DO OUR ANTIBODIES GO?

Normally when we have foreign cells or substances in our bodies, the antibodies know where to go to control the invasion. The soldiers are very smart. They usually know exactly where to go to destroy the enemy. If an infection results despite the attempts of the antibodies to fight the germs, medications can be used to control it and to help the body return to a healthy state. This could be analogous to saying that the soldiers have called in reinforcements, specialists to help deal with a specific problem that the soldiers can't handle themselves. However, in lupus, inflammations occur randomly, with no apparently predictable pattern of direction. It is not understood why these occasional inflammatory attacks occur. It is almost as if the soldiers have lost the ability to control their behavior. They go crazy and they attack wherever it is convenient for them.

In lupus, tissue damage can occur in two major ways. First, the antibodies fighting a tissue can damage it directly. For example, antibodies attacking red blood cells can destroy those cells. The second way damage occurs is from an inflammatory reaction resulting from the presence of immune complexes. What causes this? When an antibody in the blood mixes with the substances it is fighting, an immune complex is formed. Normally, the body eliminates this immune complex. However, in individuals with lupus, it is not eliminated normally and it may be trapped in certain parts of the body. This causes an inflammatory reaction that is, among other things, primarily responsible for kidney disease in people with lupus, perhaps because the kidney cannot filter out the substances. Damage from this type of inflammatory reaction can occur in other areas of the body as well. Once the immune complexes have been trapped, they trigger a sequence of events in which the body is actually trying to eliminate them, but can't. Unfortunately, in this process, the tissue in which the complexes are trapped also becomes damaged.

Inflammation resulting from the immune complexes can also occur in the connective tissues. The connective tissue, made up of a protein substance called collagen as well as fibers and supporting tissues, is the tissue that binds or connects the cells and tissues of the body together. There are connective tissues found in all parts or systems of the body. Therefore, any part of the body or any connective tissue in the body can be affected by lupus. Systemic lupus can affect virtually any organ in the body, including the heart, kidneys, brain, skin, joints, and lungs, among others. That's why the term "systemic" (meaning throughout the body) is used.

Recently, research has focused on the role of certain important white blood cells. One type of white blood cell, the B-lymphocytes, manufactures antibodies. Other white blood cells, the suppressor T-cells and the helper T-cells, normally work to help control the way the B-lymphocytes do this job. But what happens if the suppressor T-cells do not work that well? That's what happens in many people with lupus. This can lead to a malfunction in the immune system in which antibodies produced by the B-lymphocytes also attack the suppressor T-cells!

WHO GETS LUPUS?

It is estimated that up to or more than 500,000 people have lupus in the United States alone. Remember, this is an estimate. But incredibly, it means that more people have lupus than some of the more well-known illnesses, such as leukemia, multiple sclerosis, or muscular dystrophy (and there are no telethons to raise money for lupus, either!). Anywhere from 5,000 to 15,000 or more new cases of lupus are diagnosed each year.

It seems as though the number of people being diagnosed with lupus is increasing. But this is probably because people are more health conscious, and are seeing their doctors more often. Also, doctors are better able to identify lupus. There has been much improvement in diagnostic testing, and there is more awareness of the disease.

Determining Factors

Lupus can occur in all races and ethnic groups, although statistics indicate a higher than average incidence in blacks, Hispanics, and Orientals in the United States. More women than men are diagnosed with lupus. However, the percentages vary depending on what report you are reading! It's generally felt that at least 80 percent of all people with lupus are women.

Age

Is age a factor in lupus? A very high percentage of individuals diagnosed with lupus are women in their childbearing years (the years between the start of menstruation and menopause). Their age at diagnosis usually ranges, therefore, from the mid-teens to the forties. Some cases of lupus do occur earlier or later than these childbearing years, but not nearly as often. It is unusual for a child younger than five to have lupus. Scientists have been investigating the fact that both before and after the childbearing years, the number of women and the number of men who get lupus are much closer. Because men at these ages are diagnosed with lupus nearly as frequently as women, researchers hope that this may lead to a better understanding of what causes lupus.

WHAT CAUSES LUPUS?

Why does lupus occur? Why does inflammation occur in random areas of the body? Why does connective tissue become inflamed? Why, why, why? Although the causes are uncertain, researchers continue to try to come up with better answers to these questions. It is this research that has shown us that lupus is an autoimmune disease. We've learned that the antibodies produced by your body's immune system are actually causing tissue damage.

Much of the research that has been carried out is highly technical, dealing with scientific theories of the causes of lupus. One theory suggests that the autoimmune problem that occurs in lupus may be triggered by a virus. In some people, scientists have found cells that look like cells which are infected with viruses. However, others disagree with this interpretation, since similar cells can be found in people without lupus, and having lupus doesn't mean you are protected from everything else. Because of the high percentages of women in childbearing years who are diagnosed with lupus, scientists are investigating the role of hormones in lupus. Still other theories are being explored all the time.

Although it is unfortunate that the causes of lupus have not yet been determined, some treatments have been developed that can markedly reduce the impact that lupus has on your body. This can help you live a longer, more healthy, productive life, and in many cases, an essentially normal life most of the time. Hopefully, as you continue to live your life, research will provide more insight into the causes of lupus and find a cure.

IS LUPUS INHERITED?

Could you have inherited lupus? Can your children inherit lupus from you? These are frightening questions. Evidence has suggested that some autoimmune diseases may have a genetic basis. However, this does not imply that lupus is a hereditary disease. Rather, a tendency toward lupus may be what is inherited. For example, there might be a history of arthritis or other kinds of autoimmune disease in your family, or other problems with the immune system may exist. This does not mean that you have inherited lupus, or that others in your family will inherit it from you.

So what's the answer? There is no clear-cut answer. It seems most likely that both genetic and environmental variables play a role in the development of lupus. Although a susceptibility to lupus may be genetically transmitted, it probably takes some kind of environmental factor to trigger the illness. Two examples of such environmental factors are ultraviolet rays (which cause sunburns) and certain drugs, and there may be many other possibilities as well.

A Little Reassurance

Confused? O.K., here's a fact that should help you feel better. Statistics show that only about 5 percent of the children of individuals with lupus develop the illness. This implies that despite the possibility of genetic transmission of susceptibility to lupus, in most cases children still will not develop the disease. For example, even in identical twins where one twin develops lupus, only in about one third of the other members of the twin pairs does lupus also develop. Clearly, genetics is not the whole story.

RIDING THE ROLLER COASTER

When discussing lupus with her physician, Susan wanted to know if the disease would always cause the extreme pain she was feeling. She was told that her pain would probably come and go because lupus is a disease that is cyclical in nature. It's like a roller coaster, with its ups and downs. It rarely remains at the same level of intensity for long periods of time. Symptoms tend to come and go. On occasion, you may feel much better, but there are other times when the disease may flare up. When you're feeling good, there is no way of knowing how long it will be until another flare occurs. When you're in the middle of a flare and not feeling good, there is no way of knowing how long it will take until you are feeling better again.

What Triggers Lupus Flares?

Although it is still not known what causes lupus, more is being learned about what can trigger a lupus flare. Your body is changing all the time. The tissues of your body may change any time you experience something very stressful. What might be stressful enough to cause a flare? Excessive fatigue, exhaustion, emotional difficulties (such as severe stress), too much exposure to sunlight, infections, certain environmental variables, environmental chemicals, certain medications, and even injury or surgery are among the many factors that could trigger a lupus flare. What are the most common triggers? The most frequent flare-provokers seem to be fatigue, where you wear yourself down and become more vulnerable, and sunburn, where your body reacts strongly. But because you are unique, it is hard to know exactly what may cause a flare for you.

What exactly happens in a flare or remission? In a flare, lupus is affecting you body more intensely. You may be experiencing more symptoms, more effects from the symptoms that you already have, or even new symptoms. Medication will be used to try to control the symptoms. When the flare begins to subside, the use of medication will gradually be tapered off. In a remission, the symptoms and signs showing that you have lupus subside, often to the point where they are no problem at all, even without medication or with minimal maintenance therapy. When you go into remission, you return to a virtually normal state of functioning, doing most or even all of the things that you used to be able to do. In addition, lab tests that are taken at that time will often be normal, although some, like the ANA (antinuclear antibody) test, may remain positive even during remission.

This flare/remission cycle may repeat itself a number of times during the course of your illness, and some individuals with lupus never go into complete remission. Their symptoms remain at a low level of intensity, controlled with medication, with occasional flares increasing the activity of the disease.

Symptoms of lupus may appear at any time. They may disappear for no apparent reason and reappear very soon in the future or after a long period of time has transpired; again, there is often no particular obvious reason for their reoccurrence. The intervals of time may range from hours or days to months or years, and symptoms may not necessarily reappear in the same form as when they last occurred.

Can You Help Jam the Trigger?

Although modern medicine does not provide us with the means to stop lupus altogether, you can help avoid or reduce the number of lupus flares you experience by being careful of what you do. Carefully protect yourself from overexposure to the sun. Try to minimize your exposure to highly stressful, anxiety-provoking situations. Try to avoid becoming overtired. Don't overdo things. Keep the possible triggers in mind, and avoid them.

Pay attention to the early warning signs that may indicate that a flare is on its way. One of the early warning signs is a low-grade fever for no apparent reason (usually fevers ranging from 99.5°–100.5° F when the temperature is taken in the afternoon). If you find yourself growing weaker and more fatigued, or if you have a loss of pep, this may be another early warning sign. Frequent chills may also be a warning sign. Of course, advise your doctor about the appearance of any new symptoms.

Occasionally drugs may create lupus flares. If drugs are the culprit, modifying the dosages or eliminating them completely usually gets rid of the flare as well. However, the flare may not be controlled until you have stopped using the drug for a while.

HOW SERIOUS IS LUPUS?

Any chronic disease can be serious. Does this mean that because lupus is a chronic disease, everyone with lupus has a serious case of it? No! The severity of lupus varies from being very mild (most common) to being life threatening (relatively uncommon). How serious your case of lupus is depends partly on which systems of the body are affected by the disease. Certain organ involvement—kidney, brain, and heart, for instance—can have more serious implications than others, like the skin.

Betty, a 22-year-old working woman, was very upset when she found out that she had kidney involvement from her lupus. She had heard from a friend, who had read up on the subject, that kidney involvement almost always means a very serious case of lupus, one that can be fatal. She was terrified. When she consulted her doctor, however, she was reassured that having kidney involvement did not mean that her illness would be any more serious than the mild case her friend had. Because she had been having very mild symptoms, she felt even more reassured. Before her conversation with her doctor, she was afraid that the mild symptoms she was experiencing were simply the "lull before the storm." It is important to remember that mild cases can occur even with extensive systemic involvement.

The severity of lupus is also markedly affected by how well you take care of it. Do you stay out until three o'clock in the morning three or four nights each week? Do you like to sit at the beach for hours at a time? Do you make sure that your reputation as a junk-food junkie is firmly intact? Do you take your medication when you remember to take it, rather than when you should take it? Do you call your physician only when you receive a notice asking if you have moved to another town? If you use proper health procedures to take care of yourself, take medication on schedule, and keep in close contact with your physician, you can increase the chances of lupus having a much milder impact. It is important to remember that any illness, even a mild one, can become serious if it is not taken care of properly. Results are usually good with proper treatment. Carefully discuss the severity of your lupus with your physician and the treatment program you should follow to minimize its effects.

We have discussed the fact that lupus can range from being mild to severe. In general, most individuals experience mild to moderate discomfort with occasional flare-ups of more intense lupus activity.

Is Lupus Fatal?

Lupus is a chronic disease with no known cure, which means that it can last as long as you are alive. However, it is not necessarily a progressive disease, and it is most often not fatal. If you have read books and articles stating that lupus is fatal, make sure you check the copyright dates of the books or the publication dates of the articles. You'll probably find that you're not reading current information. Recent medical advances have been able to provide better treatments, and happily, this has significantly reduced the chances of lupus being fatal. There are occasions, however, when lupus can be fatal. For the most part, this occurs when lupus seriously and destructively affects important internal organs. Estimates of the mortality rate from lupus currently are 10 percent or less, meaning that out of every 100 people with lupus, 10 or fewer may die from the illness. These statistics are much better than they used to be.

It is important to remember that even though no known cure yet exists for lupus, and even though on infrequent occasions people do die from the disease, current therapies and different treatment programs have effectively reduced the mortality rate to the point where many individuals with lupus can look forward to a full life span.

THE HISTORY OF LUPUS

Will knowing the history of lupus help you feel better? Probably not, but some people are curious about where things come from. Read on if you like. You will not be quizzed on names and dates!

Symptoms of lupus had been noticed by physicians for hundreds of years, even though the illness had not yet been named. Dermatologists were the first physicians involved with the illness, and they learned to recognize it simply by looking at the facial and scarring effects. The name, however, has been applied to the illness only since the middle of the nineteenth century. Pierre Cazenave, a French dermatologist, believed that the rashes or scarred irritations on the skin looked as if the victim had been seriously bitten by a hungry wolf. In the nineteenth century many illnesses were named according to what the symptoms looked like, so in 1851 Cazenave named the illness lupus, meaning wolf. Since the skin inflammations were red, the name was expanded to lupus erythematosus, meaning "reddish wolf," to characterize lupus by its redness. This term was used to differentiate lupus from other illnesses that also affected the skin but were infectious.

The red, bitelike patches and discoloration of the individual's skin, along with the resulting scars from these irritations, now are descriptive of but not restricted to the type of lupus called discoid lupus (also called cutaneous lupus). There will be more about discoid lupus soon.

In 1872, a dermatologist named Kaposi recognized that lupus could involve parts of the body other than the skin. In 1895, Dr. William Osler, a physician at Johns Hopkins Hospital, indicated that other organs of the body could be affected in many individuals with lupus, and skin problems were just one type of involvement. Upon realizing that other systems of the body were affected in lupus, he used the phrase systemic lupus erythematosus to differentiate it from discoid lupus, which primarily affects the skin.

TWO DIFFERENT TYPES OF LUPUS

As you have learned from this short history of lupus, there are two main different types of lupus: discoid lupus and systemic lupus. Symptoms of both types can follow the cyclical pattern of coming (flare-ups) and going (remission). Even though this book primarily deals with the subject of coping with systemic lupus, it would not be complete without providing some basic information about discoid lupus as well.

Discoid Lupus

For the most part, discoid lupus involves the skin. Other organs of the body are not affected and there are no internal symptoms. In addition, discoid lupus is considered to be a milder form of lupus—with no real threat to health. Does this mean that discoid lupus is a minor problem—something to be easily ignored? No. Discoid lupus can be painful, and in some cases, scarring can result.

The word discoid is used to describe this type of lupus because the scaly, red patches, or lesions, on the skin are somewhat rounded in shape, almost like a disc. These lesions can be patchy, blotchy, or crusty. They frequently take the classic butterfly shape, extending over the bridge of the nose to the upper parts of the cheeks below the eyes.

Discoid lupus usually affects the face and neck, and sometimes lesions appear on the upper part of the chest as well. Occasionally, there may be scaly, raised lesions on the skin of the arms, the trunk, or the legs. Lesions in discoid lupus usually occur on uncovered body parts. This does not mean, however, that you should dress yourself as a mummy; there are times when covered parts of the body get these lesions as well. The term disseminated discoid lupus describes those with lesions appearing in a generalized fashion over more of the body surface than just the face, neck, and upper chest. On infrequent occasions, the lesions can affect even the palms of the hands and the soles of the feet! It is also possible for lesions to appear on the scalp, despite the fact that these lesions may be hidden by thick hair. But when the scalp is involved, there may be a permanent loss of hair in the area, resulting in baldness in that area. Patchy lesions may also occur on the tongue, inside the mouth, or in the ears.

The cause of discoid lupus remains unknown despite a number of unproven suspicions. Although it is sometimes easy to diagnose discoid lupus simply by looking for the scaly lesions, you shouldn't jump to your own conclusions about having discoid lupus. Nor should you assume that someone else has discoid lupus simply because the person has some skin irritations! Evaluation by a physician is necessary to determine if a skin condition is discoid lupus, or if skin symptoms or inflammation is from systemic lupus.

It is very important that individuals with discoid lupus take care of lesions quickly and properly and attempt to prevent additional lesions to reduce the possibility of scarring and further development of the illness. In general, lesions usually exist for fairly short periods of time, although they can remain for days, weeks, months, or even years. In extreme cases, lesions persisting for more than twenty years have been reported. With proper care, lesions may clear up in short periods of time. However, the longer the lesions persist, the greater the chance of permanent scarring and disfigurement. The two best ways to prevent the serious disfigurement or unpleasant skin effects from discoid lupus are to use proper medications, such as corticosteroids or antimalarial drugs (your physician will guide you), and to protect yourself from the ultraviolet rays of the sun.

Marianne, aged 27, was diagnosed with discoid lupus about three months ago. However, after speaking to a friend who had systemic lupus, she became very afraid that she had a greater chance of developing systemic lupus because she already had discoid lupus. She put through an urgent telephone call to her physician. As soon as he got on the phone, she asked if it was true that people who had discoid lupus had a greater chance of developing systemic lupus. She was told emphatically that there was only a slim chance, since only about 5 percent of individuals with discoid lupus develop systemic lupus.

Systemic Lupus

Bernice, a 32-year-old divorcee, went to the doctor because she noticed a butterfly rash and a few blotches on her neck. This wouldn't have concerned her too much, but she recently had been feeling more pain in her wrists and ankles. Her physician evaluated her, and diagnosed her as having systemic lupus, the other major type of lupus. This type of lupus affects internal organs and may attack any part of the body. The severity of this particular type of lupus depends on which part or organ of the body is affected. Like discoid lupus, systemic lupus may affect the skin. But the key feature that differentiates it from discoid lupus is that other internal symptoms may also be involved. Systemic lupus can be mild, but it can become more severe if some of the more important organs of the body, such as the kidneys, brain, heart, and lungs, are affected.

Frances, a 37-year-old woman, was frantic. She had been diagnosed six months ago with systemic lupus, and had slowly begun to adjust to this chronic illness. Out of the blue, she received a telephone call from a childhood friend, who, it seemed, also had lupus. Her friend, Moaning Mona, complained that she had a very severe case of lupus, and had been bedridden for months at a time. Frantic Frances hysterically called her physician to find out if this was going to happen to her. She was advised by a very wise person, "Every patient is unique. Each patient experiences lupus differently." You can even experience symptoms differently at different times with lupus, and they do come and go. When the symptoms disappear, you are said to be in a period of remission. These periods of remission can last for days, weeks, or even months or years between flare-ups.

When Frantic Frances asked if she was going to die because of lupus, she was told that the mortality rate for lupus, which used to be high, had been significantly lowered through advances in medical treatment. Frances was also warned not to read any books on lupus that were published before the early 1970s, because so much had changed in the understanding of the disease since then. She was reminded to remain in frequent touch with her physicians. But Frances was still frantic; she was still not reassured. When she asked to be told what usually happens with people who have lupus, her physician told her that most people with systemic lupus experience most difficulty with low-grade fevers, fatigue, and occasional rashes, along with joint pain or swelling. Many people with lupus rarely experience any symptoms other than these more common ones.

WHAT ARE THE SYMPTOMS OF LUPUS?

The symptoms of lupus can be divided into several categories. No one ever has all the symptoms. Some people have some of them, but most have only a few of them.

- *General Symptoms.* Such symptoms as weakness, fatigue, low-grade fevers, generalized aching, and chills are included in this category. These symptoms are most often evident when you're in a flare, although you may experience them fairly constantly throughout the course of your illness.
- *Skin.* Skin problems include rashes, patchy lesions, and red inflammations. Scarring on the skin of the scalp may be related to hair loss. Skin rashes from exposure to sunlight may occur. Bruising occurs commonly and more easily in people with lupus.
- *Chest.* Symptoms involving the chest include chest pain due to pleurisy, an irritation of the membranes lining the inside of the chest around the lungs, and pain due to pericarditis, an inflammation of the sac surrounding the heart. With both of these manifestations, difficulty in breathing may occur and pain is common. Shortness of breath or a rapid heartbeat may also result. Inflammation in the rib area or in the abdominal muscles may cause chest pain as well.
- *Muscular System.* Symptoms involving the muscular system primarily include weakness and aching pain.
- *Joints.* Joint pain is common in lupus: arthritislike pain, swelling in the joints, redness, and stiffness. These symptoms may involve one or more joints, but the arthritis is rarely deforming in lupus.
- *Blood.* Lupus may also affect the blood. A low red blood cell count (anemia) is common in individuals with lupus, and can be one cause of fatigue. White blood cell counts may also decrease, leading to an increased susceptibility to infection. On the other hand, if there is an infection in the body, the white blood cell count may signifi-

cantly increase. Increased amounts of gamma globulin (the general name for the protein portion of the blood that contains antibodies) in the blood may also be seen with lupus, and blood tests may indicate a false positive test for syphilis. Lupus patients may test positive for syphilis even though they do not have the disease because one of the "abnormal" lupus antibodies reacts with a substance on the cell wall of the bacterium that causes syphilis.

- *Cardiac or Circulatory Involvement.* It is sometimes difficult to tell if you have cardiac involvement. You might notice increased swelling in your extremities, such as your feet, and feel shortness of breath. You may have an accumulation of fluid in the sac surrounding your heart. Cardiac involvement can be dangerous but does clear up when treatment is effective. The most common circulatory problem is Raynaud's phenomenon, in which spasms in the small blood vessels restrict the flow of blood to the extremities.

- *Digestive System Involvement.* Stomach pain, cramps, nausea, vomiting, diarrhea, and constipation are occasional symptoms of lupus occurring in the digestive tract.

- *Kidney Involvement.* Your kidneys may be less efficient in filtering waste out of the blood. Waste products remain in circulation, and uremia (an increase in waste products in the blood) may occur. In addition, there may be excessive amounts of protein lost in the urine, a condition called proteinuria. Since there is no pain associated with these changes, it is important to see your physician regularly so you can be tested for abnormal kidney function.

- *Nervous System Involvement.* Various parts of the nervous system including the brain, spinal cord, and nerves may be involved. This may result in headaches or, in more severe cases, in symptoms such as seizures, temporary paralysis, or psychotic behavior, or even strokes.

There are many symptoms of lupus. You may have only one or you may have several. You may have the same ones all the time, or they may change. Who knows what will happen? The only sure thing about lupus is that there is no sure thing about lupus!

IS LUPUS CONTAGIOUS?

One of Susan's primary concerns when she was first told that she had lupus was that she would be unable to stay with her husband and children or they would catch her disease. Many people who are newly diagnosed with lupus are concerned that lupus may be contagious. This is also a major concern of friends and relatives who do not know anything about the illness. Because lupus sounds frightening, "friends" may be very concerned about being with you because of their fear of catching it from you. There has never been a documented case of anyone catching lupus! Since lupus is far from a rare disease, if it were contagious, such cases would certainly have been reported by now. And how about physicians? Wouldn't they be at risk if lupus were contagious? Be assured that physicians are no more likely to have lupus than anybody else. So, Susan, wherever you are, lupus is not contagious. You need not be concerned about anybody catching it from you, so don't be afraid to be with anyone.

2

How Is Lupus Diagnosed?

After Susan got over her initial shock from being diagnosed with lupus, she asked her doctor to explain how he had finally concluded that she had the disease. He told her about the difficulties physicians have in accurately diagnosing lupus. As a matter of fact, he marvelled at the fact that all physicians trying to diagnose lupus were not bald from pulling their hair out in frustration!

THE PROBLEMS IN DIAGNOSIS

It is shocking that it can take several years for someone to be diagnosed with lupus. Several years! This doesn't mean that it takes that long for you to drag your symptom-laden body to the doctor! Because the initial symptoms of lupus may not be very noticeable or serious, you may not be inclined to go to the doctor to have them checked out. As the symptoms worsen and you are more aware of your fatigue and joint pain, you may then decide to go to the doctor. As you have the disease for longer periods of time, more symptoms of lupus may occur. (Remember, you're not involved in any treatment program yet.) This can make the eventual diagnosis easier because the package of symptoms will paint a picture for the diagnosing physician. But if your doctor doesn't come up with the right diagnosis, or if you run out of patience, you may end up going from doctor to doctor, trying different medications and treatments until you finally get the proper diagnosis or the correct treatment.

Lupus has frequently been called the great imitator. There is an incredible number of symptoms you can have with lupus. Therefore,

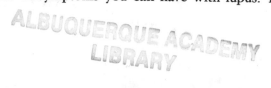

physicians who are trying to diagnose you may initially believe that another illness is the problem. Treatment may be started for the other illness. Only after seeing that the symptoms continue unabated may further investigation take place. Hopefully, trial and error will eventually result in the correct diagnosis of lupus.

What else makes it hard to diagnose lupus, especially in its early stages? Laboratory tests used to diagnose illnesses are not always correct. In a small percentage of cases, the findings are totally wrong! The tests may show no existence of lupus in someone who, using other criteria, has been diagnosed with lupus. This is called a false negative (the test saying, "No, you don't have it," when you really do). On the other hand, some people who do not have lupus will show a weak, but nevertheless existing, positive lupus reaction to some of these blood tests. This is called a false positive (the test saying, "You have it," when you really don't). Lab tests are only suggestive. Your whole medical history is most important in diagnosing lupus. Therefore, it is very important for you to have a wise, informed, and concerned doctor.

Researchers are still trying to come up with the perfect lab test for lupus. Maybe someday . . .

SETTING UP DIAGNOSTIC CRITERIA

You can now understand how difficult it is for physicians to diagnose lupus. Of course, that may not make you feel better. So what can be done to make a correct diagnosis of lupus? If lupus mimics other diseases, and laboratory tests for it are sometimes inaccurate, how do physicians ever determine if anyone has lupus? After a lot of deliberation and analysis, fourteen criteria for lupus were established in 1971 by the American Rheumatism Association. Physicians generally agreed that it was likely that you had lupus if you had a positive response to four or more of the fourteen criteria for lupus.

Our understanding of lupus is constantly changing. When the initial manuscript for the first edition of this book was written, physicians were still following the fourteen criteria. By the time the final revisions were being completed, the criteria had been condensed to a revised list of eleven items.

Will these eleven items occur only in a person who has lupus? No. Anyone could have a positive response to an item, so satisfying any one particular criterion certainly does not mean you have lupus. That is why at least four of the criteria must occur. As you read through the criteria, see which items apply to you.

THE ELEVEN CRITERIA

A patient should meet *at least four* of the following eleven criteria to be diagnosed with lupus:

1. Facial redness or a rash on the face. This frequently appears in the form of the butterfly configuration. The rash may be on both sides of the face, or just on one side. It is usually flat.
2. A more extensive skin problem that may show as a rash, blotches, or raised scaly lesions. Scarring may result. These thick, raised patches are shaped somewhat like discs, and may occur on any part of the body. This is the main symptom of discoid lupus.
3. Photosensitivity. This means that the individual has some kind of harmful physiological reaction to sunlight—more severe than just a sunburn! Many people aside from those having lupus are sensitive to sunlight, especially those with fair complexions. So, in order to meet this criterion, your reaction should be significant, even with minimal exposure to sunlight.
4. The existence of ulcers (sores) in either the mouth or nose, or the throat. Although many people have had sores in their mouths from time to time, how often these sores occur is relevant in lupus.
5. Arthritislike symptoms in two or more joints. Arthritic inflammation or pain must not be accompanied by any noticeable or marked deformity of these joints to meet this criterion. Arthritic problems in a joint show up as swelling or tenderness, or pain if the joint is moved. The joints that may be affected include the feet, ankles, fingers, knees, hips, elbows, shoulders, wrists, and jaw.
6. Your having either pericarditis or pleurisy. Pericarditis is an inflammation of the sac or lining surrounding the heart, and pleurisy involves inflammation of the membrane that lines the inside of the chest cavity surrounding the lungs. Both conditions can be painful. Your having either of these two conditions meets the requirement for this criterion.
7. Your having one of two possible kidney problems. One is the existence of excessive protein in the urine. This is called pro-

teinuria. The other is the existence of blood cell "casts." These are fragments of cells normally found in the blood. If you have kidney disease, however, they may be found in the urine. The seventh criterion is met if either of these two problems occur.

8. Occurrence of a neurological disorder, either convulsions (seizures) or psychotic behavior, without it possibly being caused by drugs or a metabolic problem.

9. Specific changes in the blood (blood disorders). One blood problem that can occur with lupus is hemolytic anemia. Anemia is a common blood disorder. But if you have hemolytic anemia (where the red cells are coated with antibodies that cause them to break down and break apart), it may indicate that you have lupus. It is important to remember that red blood cells normally live, die, and are eliminated naturally. In hemolytic anemia the blood cells are destroyed because of this antibody coating, and so they are eliminated too rapidly and prematurely.

    A second potential problem with the blood may be a low white blood count resulting from destruction of your white blood cells. This condition is called leukopenia. Since individuals with lupus frequently do have a low white blood count, this is an important criterion for diagnosis of lupus even if it occurs early in the disease. White blood cells fight infection in the body.

    A third blood disorder is lymphopenia, where there is a decrease in the number of lymphocytes (types of white blood cells) in the blood. Lymphocytes are the main cells of the immune system.

    The leukopenia and lymphopenia must be detected on two or more occasions for this to be one of the criteria in the diagnosis of lupus.

    A fourth type of problem with the blood is called thrombocytopenia, which is a problem with the platelets in the blood. You may have trouble forming blood clots if you get a cut or a wound. Therefore, the bleeding may be more difficult to control. Thrombocytopenia must be detected in the absence of any medicine known to cause this problem.

10. A disorder in your immune system. One possibility might be the presence of the LE cell. The LE (lupus erythematosus) cell contains two nuclei rather than the one nucleus that cells usually have. Two nuclei are present in the LE cell because people with lupus have antibodies in their blood that can "bind" with the

nuclei of cells. When the antibodies bind with nuclei, they increase the likelihood that a scavenger cell will ingest this antibody-coated nucleus. So the cell with two nuclei is simply a cell that has its own nucleus along with a second nucleus that it has ingested because of the antibody coating the second nucleus.

LE cells are found in about 60 percent of all people who have lupus, especially when the disease is in a flare phase. At the same time, LE cells are rarely found if you don't have lupus. So the presence of LE cells is an important indicator. In order for this criterion to be met, lab tests should show two or more LE cells on any particular occasion, or one LE cell should be microscopically observed on two or more occasions. However, in many centers this test is not being used, primarily because it is difficult to do accurately, and it is very time consuming. Besides, as mentioned above, over one third of all individuals with lupus would not show a positive result anyway.

Another way of satisfying the tenth criterion is to obtain a false positive reaction to the test for syphilis. The reason that this item is included in the list is because of the frequency with which individuals with lupus do show this false positive reaction to the test for syphilis. If the test for syphilis does come back positive, additional tests should be used to make sure that syphilis really doesn't exist. Some may be embarrassed because they have a positive reaction to a syphilis test. But laboratory tests can distinguish between a false positive result due to one of the abnormal lupus antibodies and a real case of syphilis, so it is an important diagnostic test.

11. The production of antinuclear antibodies (ANA). Instead of fighting the foreign invaders that cause disease in the body, these antibodies actually turn against the nuclei of good healthy cells. Because many individuals with lupus do produce antinuclear antibodies, a positive result to the ANA test may help to diagnose the illness.

Evaluating the Criteria

So, how many criteria did you meet? Remember, any *one* of the above criteria may exist in anyone, with or without lupus. It is the *combination* of the criteria and the severity and duration of a symptom that may help determine whether or not you have lupus.

Although they are currently the best accepted guidelines, these criteria are not unchallenged. Some physicians feel that this list is not comprehensive enough, or that there are still some important factors that have been left out. Some items on the list are not considered to be as important as other items on the list. Some physicians question whether certain items should be included at all. More revisions of the list will undoubtedly be seen in the future.

Another criticism of the established criteria is the requirement that four of the eleven be met. What if you clearly have been suffering from the symptoms of lupus, but meet fewer than four criteria? Does this mean you don't have lupus? No. What if you meet four or more of the criteria? Does this definitely guarantee that you have lupus? No. Obviously, these are valid criticisms. Not all cases will be diagnosed correctly. But when used properly, the criteria at least increase the chance for an accurate diagnosis.

Remember: A proper diagnosis of systemic lupus is made after careful consideration of your medical history, a detailed physical examination, and an assessment of appropriate laboratory test results.

3

How Is Lupus Treated?

So far, we have discussed what lupus is, who may get it, what some of the symptoms of lupus are, and what criteria may be used to diagnose the illness, as well as other details about the disease. Terrific, but you're probably less concerned about what it is and where it came from than you are about how you can feel better. True? You probably have some important questions. What can your doctors do for you? What will doctors tell you to do? What is the treatment for lupus and how will it affect you? How do you control your symptoms? How do you help yourself get back into the mainstream of life? Let's begin to answer some of the questions about the treatment of lupus.

YOUR ROLE IN TREATMENT

There are always things you can do to help yourself. It doesn't matter how much medical knowledge you have. There are also things you can do that will make your condition worse, but obviously those are things to be avoided. To start helping yourself, identify those things that improve your condition and those things that hurt it.

Physicians can provide much in the way of medical information, medication, and expertise. Family and friends can provide emotional support, caring, and guidance. But you are the only one who can make the many small decisions necessary to organize your lifestyle as much as possible. These decisions may be small, but they may be critical in determining how lupus affects you. Therefore, it is obvious that you can play an important role in influencing the way you feel. But that's not enough. No single factor is enough. To help yourself best, a whole package approach is essential, where you help yourself in as many ways as possible, both medically and psychologically.

THE GOAL OF TREATMENT

Because there is no known cure for lupus, treatment ideally aims at a suppression of symptoms. You want to feel better, right? Well, that's the goal of treatment, along with protecting and strengthening your body. You want to reduce the impact of your symptoms. However, this is not the ideal outcome. The ideal outcome is remission, where symptoms no longer exist. Although your active treatment of lupus with medication and lifestyle changes aims to suppress symptoms, hopefully these symptoms will completely disappear and you'll go into remission.

INDIVIDUALIZED TREATMENT

Your experience with lupus is unique. No one else has the same set of symptoms or reactions to the disease. At the same time, each physician who sets up a treatment program for someone will put together a unique package based on the needs of the person being treated.

Each physician usually has his or her own idea as to what types of treatments work best. If you went to five different physicians and described the same symptoms to each, each of the five physicians might well prescribe a different treatment program for you. There may be no one specific approach that is right. A lot of trial and error goes into developing the best treatment program for you, and you may feel like a human guinea pig. But remember, this is only because the goal is to find the package that works best for you. Because of the number of unknowns concerning lupus and how it affects you, it may take some time before your physicians find the best way to treat you. Because there is no absolute treatment, modifications may be necessary before your treatment program works best. Does that mean that there aren't any physicians who agree on how lupus should be treated? No. There is a lot of agreement. Most physicians do prescribe a similar treatment program for their patients, adjusting it appropriately for you as an individual.

It is very important for you to feel at ease with your physician. You want to have confidence in the treatment program prescribed for you. What if you heard that somebody else with lupus was receiving different treatment from a different physician, and you started to believe that the other treatment program might be better. You might start losing confidence in your treatment plan, and then in your own physician. Not a great feeling, is it? Remember, there is no one answer! What works for somebody else will not necessarily work for you.

Rarely will your treatment program remain constant throughout the course of your illness. If your symptoms become more pronounced or severe (let's hope not), treatment programs may become more active and intensified. If your symptoms become less intense, the treatment programs may become less active and more relaxed.

What are your symptoms? Treatment will be aimed at the symptoms that are specifically affecting you. Frequently, carefully structured treatment programs can be successful in controlling symptoms to the point where you can really be yourself. However, there are times when the treatment program is not able to reduce all symptoms. Medications or other therapies may not successfully control a symptom of lupus in one particular part of the body or another, or complications may arise. But you'll work with your physician, and you'll cross that bridge if and when you come to it.

If you are in a flare, think about what may have caused it. If you are doing something that gets you sick every time you do it, then stop doing it! For example, consider sunbathing (or maybe you shouldn't consider it!). Let's say that every time you go out in the sun, within a day or even a few hours after exposure you get a rash and a fever. Part of your treatment, therefore, should include restricting your exposure to sunlight and using a sunblock lotion.

CAN YOU PREDICT THE FUTURE COURSE
OF THE ILLNESS?

Despite the fact that treatment for lupus has been more and more successful, it is impossible to predict the future course of your illness. It still is not known what leads to a remission, how long any remission will last, or whether you will ever be symptom free. What other reasons are there for the difficulty in predicting the future course of your condition? Lupus is never a constant illness; it is always changing. Different systems and organs can be affected. Your age and attentiveness to your treatment program may also play a role in the severity of the disease.

Programs will change as symptoms decrease in intensity or other symptoms occur. This requires that you work in partnership with your physician. Let the physician know of any changes in symptoms, whether they're better or worse, so that treatment is changed accordingly. Never change your treatment on your own.

TREATMENT COMPONENTS:
A GENERAL CONSENSUS

Professionals involved with the treatment of lupus recognize that the best, most effective treatment program incorporates four major components: (1) adjustment of general lifestyle, involving changes in behavior and activity necessitated by lupus; (2) coping with emotional reactions, because it is so important that stress and negative emotions be controlled to avoid further problems with your health; (3) proper medication, which plays such a major role in suppression of symptoms; and (4) attention to diet and nutritional needs. Each of these components will be discussed in detail in subsequent chapters.

PART II
Your Emotions

4

Coping With Your Emotions— An Introduction

How unhappy are you about having lupus? Well, each person's emotional responses to lupus are different. Even your own reactions to lupus will vary from time to time. The more severe your reactions are, the more these will interfere with your ability to cope.

Your emotions can ride the roller coaster just like lupus does. As a matter of fact, emotional ups and downs are very common. It is estimated that far more than half of all people with lupus experience emotional problems because of their illness. Your emotional reactions to lupus may start even before treatment has begun. Of course, your reaction will also depend on how suddenly your condition developed. For example, if your condition seemed to appear almost overnight, you might not adjust as well as if it developed slowly.

When first diagnosed, some people may not react at all, since their condition still may not be "real" to them. But others go through a hard time. You may know someone who has lupus, or have heard about somebody's experiences with lupus. Perhaps this frightened you. Emotional reactions to lupus are not always rational. As a matter of fact, in many cases they are completely irrational. As the full impact of the diagnosis sets in, you may experience a whole variety of emotional reactions, ranging from sadness and anxiety to anger, frustration, and despair.

FACTORS SHAPING YOUR EMOTIONAL REACTIONS

A number of factors may play a role in determining how you react to lupus. Keep in mind, however, that because there are so many factors, no one can predict how a person will react at any given time. How did you handle problems before your condition was diagnosed? What was your general coping style? Were you calm or nervous? Were you persistent or did you give up easily? The way you handle life's problems in general will indicate how well you will cope with lupus and its treatment.

Are you successful in coping with stress? The stress of having lupus is partly related to how lupus came about, how long each flare or remission lasts, how intense the symptoms are, and what kind of treatment you need, among other factors.

Your age has a bearing on how you respond emotionally. Your general physical health prior to the onset of lupus also plays a role in determining your coping ability. What about your relationships? In many cases, your emotional reactions may reflect the responses of loved ones and close friends. For example, your reactions may be affected by family members or friends who are anxious about your medical condition. And if there is any central nervous system involvement, there may be organic, physiological causes for emotional disturbances.

WHAT EMOTIONAL PROBLEMS CAN OCCUR FROM LUPUS?

Have you ever felt intense anger because you have to go through all this? Are you angry that your life will change because of lupus? Are you afraid of the medication you may need? Do you become depressed when you compare your present life to the way things were? Are you afraid that you won't be able to cope? Do you fear facing a bleak, if not hopeless, future? Some of the most common emotional reactions to lupus are depression, fear, guilt, and anger. Because of the importance of coping with these emotions, a separate chapter has been devoted to each of them. But other than these specific emotional responses, what else might you experience?

Do you like yourself less since your diagnosis? Previous feelings of confidence can be quickly shattered. Loss of self-esteem can have a very unpleasant effect on you. You may not feel or behave the way you used to. You'll want to deal with this right away in order to return to effective, efficient functioning.

You may feel disoriented. Do you sometimes feel that things around you are unreal? One of the most frightening feelings is that you're not yourself, especially if you don't know why you're feeling this way. It can be reassuring to understand that these episodes do occur from time to time, both because of lupus activity and because of medication, such as steroids, that you may be taking. It is helpful to be aware of these effects, and to know that by just riding them out, or by changing medication dosages, these episodes will go away.

How about mood swings? Do you ever experience these? Many individuals with lupus do. You may be concerned that your mood swings are caused by the illness. But if you stop to think about it, we all experience mood swings from time to time, whether we have lupus or not! It is possible that medication, especially high dosages of steroids, can increase the range of these mood swings. But let your physician know what's going on, so changes can be made.

MANAGING EMOTIONAL REACTIONS

Some of the ways people have adjusted to lupus and its treatment have included therapeutic intervention, support groups, and education. Because your emotions play such an important role in life with lupus, you'll certainly want to do the best possible job of controlling them. How? Let's discuss some of the more important ways.

Medical Management

Make sure you're getting the best possible medical care. If you haven't already done so, you'll want to establish a good working relationship with your physician. This involves seeing a doctor who not only has expertise in treating lupus, but is also understanding, available, and sympathetic to your emotional needs. You'll want to be sure that your physician watches your condition carefully, so any problems that may arise can be caught early. Your physician must also monitor your dosages of medication carefully, so that they are used most effectively and so that any side effects are minimized.

Support Groups

Joining a self-help or support group can be very enlightening. You'll see how others handle problems, some of which may be the same as or at least similar to your own. Groups provide a forum for the exchange of feelings and ideas, as well as suggestions on how to cope better. You'll see that you're not alone. This is probably the most important reason for belonging to a group.

These groups are also wonderful for your family, giving family members the chance to get some support of their own. Since one of the best ways to be in control of your emotions is to have a supportive family behind you, you should encourage their participation, too.

Do you ever feel shunned or ignored by others, or do you fear feeling this way? Are your social relationships dwindling? Groups can give you a feeling of belonging. There are people that you can be with—people who share a common bond—because they, too, are living with lupus.

In groups, any topics you'd like to talk about can be discussed. You may begin to share feelings more openly when you hear others talking about subjects you were previously reluctant to bring up yourself. As a result, a feeling of closeness—almost like family—develops.

Many times, members of groups dealing with chronic illnesses discuss feelings of hostility toward the medical profession. A person alone with these feelings may have a hard time dealing with physicians and trusting them. Talking about these feelings in a group can hopefully straighten them out so that a more positive, constructive relationship with a medical professional can be formed.

The most important purpose of belonging to a group, however, is the sharing of ideas design to help you cope. Methods of coping and techniques for helping yourself feel better are shared, suggestions are offered, and social relationships can develop.

Belonging to a national organization, such as the Lupus Foundation of America or The American Lupus Society, can be helpful. Such organizations bring patients and families together, and provide lots of beneficial information. They also help to expand public awareness of lupus and its treatment. This will also help you with your emotions, since the more people who understand what's involved with lupus, the less alone and isolated you'll feel.

By the way, there's no law that says that emotional reactions *have* to be shared with others. It's not necessary to talk about them, even though this can be helpful. But these emotional reactions do need to be recognized and worked through. That's the only way to make progress.

Medication

You'll frequently hear about medications that improve depression, anxiety, anger, and other emotional problems. Medication prescribed for these purposes is usually not addictive, so you might not be as reluctant to take it. Antianxiety medication can be helpful. So can mood elevators and antidepressants. But just remember that your doctor is the one who is in charge of medication. Don't "play with fire."

Psychological Strategies

Professional intervention may be necessary if your emotional problems are severe, or if you want to prevent them from getting worse. Having somebody to talk to can be a big help, especially with an illness like lupus, which has its ups and downs. Of course, there are some things *you* can do about your emotions.

HELPING YOURSELF

Let's discuss some of the best techniques you can use to improve the way you feel.

Laugh a Little

Humor can be an amusingly effective way to deal with emotions. Whether it is hearing a joke from someone else, laughing at yourself, or creating your own jokes, humor can be a very relaxing way of dealing with a troublesome situation.

Humor works in three ways. First of all, it reduces anxiety. Laughing is a great way to release tension. Second, it can distract you from those things or feelings that are bothering you. When you're involved in something humorous, you often feel a lot better. Think back, for example, to a time when you were depressed or uncomfortable and somebody asked if you had heard a certain joke. Initially you may have been reluctant to hear it. But before long you were probably totally absorbed in the joke, wondering what the punch line would be! The fact that humor can distract you also means that it can help you to see things from a different perspective. So you may be able to look at something more objectively, which can help you to handle it more effectively.

Finally, the ability to laugh at yourself is a helpful coping strategy. It's also an important part of maturing. How well this works, however, depends on what you're going through. It's just about impossible (and probably ridiculous) to laugh at yourself while you're going through a crisis. However, as you adjust to your condition, you can better use humor as a coping strategy.

Relaxation Procedures

Relaxation is the opposite of tension. So if you learn to relax, you'll be much less tense. But relaxation procedures by themselves will not totally control your emotions. So why use them? Because if you're feeling more relaxed, you'll be better able to identify those problems that are affecting you, and you'll then be better able to figure out how to deal with them. Relaxation procedures, then, can be an essential first step in coping with your emotions.

How do you relax? We're talking about clinical relaxation, now— not everyday activities like reading, gardening, listening to music, or sitting in front of the television with a can of beer! There are different types of clinical relaxation procedures. For example, progressive relaxation is a procedure in which you learn how to relax the muscles in your body. Hypnosis is another relaxation procedure, as are meditation and the relaxation response. There's also a procedure called imagery, in which you view pictures in your mind to help you relax, thereby making it easier for you to solve problems. (More information about imagery can be found in Chapter 14, "Pain.") Books on any of these procedures are available in your local library, and can really help you to start feeling better.

Here's a quick introduction to one relaxation procedure. I call it, appropriately, the "quick release." Read the directions first and then try it. Close your eyes, take a deep breath, and hold it as you tighten every muscle in your body that you can think of—your fists, arms, legs, stomach, neck, buttocks, etc. Hold your breath, keeping your muscles tense, for about six seconds. Then let it out in a "whoosh," and allow the tension to drain out of your muscles. Let your body go limp. Keep your eyes closed, and breathe rhythmically and comfortably for about twenty seconds. Repeat this tension-relaxation cycle three times. By the end of the third repetition, you'll probably feel a lot more relaxed.

Pinpointing

Are you more comfortable now? Then you're ready to proceed to the next crucial step. In order to deal with anything that's upsetting you,

you'll want to determine exactly what it is that's bothering you! Make a list of these things. Then go over what you've written. In reviewing your list, you'll see that just about every item can be placed into one of two categories. The first category contains the modifiables, or the things (whether problems or emotions) you *can* do something about. The second category includes the nonmodifiables, or the things you *can't* do anything about. Why separate them? Because you should take two different courses of action to deal with each.

For the first category, you'll want to figure out what strategies you can use to improve the situation. You can plan a course of action as soon as you identify exactly what's bothering you. How about the second category? You'll still be planning strategies, but of a different kind! Where do your emotions exist? In your mind, right? Therefore, your plan for this category is to work on the way you're thinking.

What Should You Do?

How can you change your thinking so that something will bother you less? The technique you use really depends on what emotional reaction is bothering you. For example, if you're afraid of something and you want to conquer this fear, a procedure called systematic desensitization may be helpful. We'll go into this later in Chapter 7, "Fears and Anxieties."

If you're feeling guilty or angry about something, or if something is depressing you, it can be very helpful for you to learn how to change or "restructure" the way you're thinking. You'll learn more about techniques for that in Chapters 6, 8, and 9.

Actually, any of the procedures we've discussed can be used with just about any problem. It's just a question of deciding what's best for *you* in how you cope with your emotions.

WHAT ABOUT THE FUTURE?

Even if you do have intense emotional reactions, these will diminish either because of the passage of time or because you're doing something to help. On the other hand, you'll experience more emotional reactions when your symptoms are more pronounced. So you'll probably experience a range of emotional reactions from time to time. But even when these feelings do occur, you can usually point to so many positive things going on in your life—so many areas in which you can recognize progress—that it may not be such a difficult thing to deal with.

Although emotions do not cause lupus, they can certainly interfere with your ability to live with the disease. In addition, emotional upsets can, in some cases, exacerbate your condition. So doesn't it make sense to do what you can to control your emotions?

The purpose of this section is to help you understand the different emotions you may experience. You'll discover where they come from and, very importantly, recognize that many others have gone through exactly what you're going through. In addition, a number of strategies will be presented to help you cope with these emotions more effectively. Remember that "practice makes better." (There's no such thing as perfect.) Just reading about a method to control an emotion doesn't mean you'll experience instant success. You have to keep practicing.

In the following chapters you'll see how these different techniques can be used. So don't be afraid, depressed, guilty, or angry! Instead, read on!

5

Coping With the Diagnosis

When you first found out that you had lupus, how did you feel? How did you react when your doctor finally told you the news? In all probability, you experienced one of several different types of reactions.

YOU MIGHT BE RELIEVED!

One type of reaction is that of relief. Now that may seem strange to you! Why would you be relieved to know that you have lupus? Well, perhaps you've been experiencing a lot of pain and nothing's seemed to help. Or maybe you've tried to get a diagnosis for a long time. Amazingly, research has shown that it can take years to diagnose lupus in some people. That's a very long time for you to wonder what's wrong, especially considering how sick you've been feeling. It may have been particularly hard on you if you looked O.K. and the people close to you couldn't understand why you were so tired. You've been sick for so long, and you've endured different symptoms. You've gone from doctor to doctor, trying to find out what was really wrong with you, so you could begin a treatment plan that would finally help you feel better. Maybe physicians or your family and friends didn't believe you were really ill, and thought the problem was all in your head! That could really be annoying! If things went on indefinitely as they had been, you may have started wondering yourself!

You might have thought you had cancer or some other fatal illness. (Some people actually feel this way!) Certain symptoms may have really frightened you. Wow, were you relieved to find out that you weren't dying! So knowing what the cause is can be a relief.

At last, the correct diagnosis is made. If you were relieved after your diagnosis, you probably had a much easier time coping with the start of treatment. Why? One reason is because you're hopeful that treatment will significantly improve the way you've been feeling (and it's good to finally know *why* you're feeling that way). Second, family members and friends who may not have believed that you were really sick will now discover the truth. Unfortunately, some people close to you may still not believe that the problem is physical. They may continue to believe that the problem is either emotional or stress related. You can't make everyone believe a medical diagnosis! However, most doubts will probably disappear. Strained relationships may improve. Family members may sometimes feel guilty as they realize that they have been skeptical about your condition. They may have criticized your inability to fulfill responsibilities and your decreased ability to do things. They did this because they thought a real illness did not exist. Now they know the truth! Third, and most important, you'll be relieved that it wasn't all in your head. After a long period of time, even the most confident person may have begun to wonder whether or not there was really something wrong or if the problem was purely emotional.

YOU MAY PANIC!

The other less pleasant reaction is one of terror. Sheer panic! You might have reacted, "Oh, no, I have lupus! What is it? Where does it come from? Why do I have it?" or thought, "I'm too young for this!" Or you may ask, "What's going to happen to me?" "How will the disease affect me?" "Will I ever be 'normal'?" "What is the treatment and how will I handle it?" "Am I going to be confined to a wheelchair?" "Will I ever get better?" "Who will take care of me?" "Am I going to die?" These are all tense questions that may pop up when you're diagnosed. Family members and loved ones may ask them (and panic) as well. You may think that your life may never be the same again, for life will now include treatment for lupus.

Let's talk about this reaction. Nobody enjoys pain or physical restrictions. It's normal to be afraid. You probably don't understand the diagnosis. (Not many diagnosed with lupus knew about the illness beforehand.) After all, lupus even sounds frightening! You may suddenly be hit with the fact that you are mortal and vulnerable. You'll realize you may have this problem for the rest of your life. It's not uncommon to feel faint or to experience a shortness of breath or other stress reactions at the time of diagnosis.

YOU MIGHT FEEL CALM!

Frequently, as with any traumatic event, you may feel numb at first. You may sit quietly in the doctor's office, listening to everything that is being said. But you may not really be absorbing it. You may hear your doctor talking, but his words are not penetrating. You might even actively and calmly participate in the discussion without any emotional reaction. That may come later!

HOW ABOUT DENIAL?

Denying that a problem exists is not unusual. Regardless of what symptoms you've been experiencing, hearing that you have lupus may provoke denial. You may protest, "Oh, you're just making that up," "I don't have this problem the way you think I do," "Why don't you give it a little more time? I'm sure the problem will go away by itself," or even "#!(*) x#, leave me alone!"

If you're reading this book, then chances are you're probably not denying your condition. But if you are denying it, the best way to start coping with your situation is to face reality. Speak to those professionals who know about your condition and have them explain it in further detail. Let them explain why treatment is necessary. Look at any X-rays that have been taken. Talk to other people with lupus and listen to what they went through when they were first diagnosed. You will find that many of their experiences parallel your own. You may also discover self-help groups that can add to your knowledge of lupus, as well as your coping ability.

Did you ever ask yourself, "Why can't things go back to the way they used to be?" Have you ever wished you could wake up one morning and find out that this was all a bad dream? The more you keep hoping that your illness will go away, the more you are slowing down your adjustment. Why is this so? Because you're not admitting to yourself that you've changed—perhaps permanently. Instead of facing the truth, you're trying to push it out of your mind, hoping that things will return to the way they were. Such denial can obviously make it hard to cope with having lupus, since the problem is not being faced realistically. Try to recognize that your condition does exist now, that it affects you, and that it will remain with you. Try to plan all your activities and aim all your thinking toward the notion that you are going to do what you can to handle it effectively.

DEATH WISH

Did you ever wish you could die after being told you have lupus? Some people do. Emotionally, they exclaim that they'd rather die than have to go through this,. If you've ever felt this way, don't feel guilty about such thoughts. You're not alone. Although you may feel like giving up from time to time, these feelings can go away if you work hard enough on them.

HOW DO YOU START TO ADJUST?

You must help yourself. Although you may have the love and support of family and friends, and your physicians may offer their guidance and expertise, it's not enough. *You* are the one who is going to have to come to grips with your condition. This is something you have to do yourself, regardless of what anyone else says or does. At first, adjusting may be a very difficult and ongoing struggle. It may require a lot of effort and understanding. You may go through a lot of emotional turmoil, but there is no other way to deal with your illness successfully. You must face it.

Information, please! Get as much of it as you can. Most of your initial reactions probably occurred because you didn't know enough about lupus. So you'll want to learn as much as possible. Your physician will be helpful in providing information, or will at least suggest ways of getting it. Read a lot, but make sure that your reading material is current. Check to make sure the information is not outdated. Not only can older books and magazines—more than five years old, let's say—be misleading, but they can be downright dangerous and depressing. Many times people have been devastated because they read old information giving very little hope for a happy life with lupus.

After reading general, consumer-oriented information, you might want to move on to more technical material. Ask questions about anything you don't understand. It probably wasn't a lifelong goal of yours to become an expert on lupus, but think about how much this can help you. Doctors will respect your questions more. And you'll understand exactly what's going on in your body. These are just two of the many advantages that can come from reading about your condition.

Support services and organizations such as the Lupus Foundation of America have the specific purpose of providing you with current information on lupus. Not only do these organizations have reading material, but they often sponsor forums, symposia, speakers, groups, and self-help classes all designed to help you.

Beware of Less Reputable Sources

Should you believe everything you read? Of course not. You may come across "cures" in weekly newspapers or magazines that sound incredible—alternatives for proper treatment that make you regret having started it in the first place. Or you may read in a glossy, weekly magazine that snake venom was successful in eliminating all lupus symptoms! (Don't count on it!) Make sure that whatever you read is reputable, and remember that it takes rigorous scientific study before one can prove that a new procedure or treatment is actually effective. And be sensible. If some exciting new treatment or medication was discovered, wouldn't you expect to learn about it in your daily newspaper or on a national news program? More about this later in Chapter 21, "Quackery."

DEALING WITH YOUR EMOTIONAL REACTIONS

Begin working consciously to control any anxiety or stress that's making you feel less than comfortable. Once you have accepted the fact that you have a chronic illness and have to alter your lifestyle, you'll want to try to control as many harmful emotions as you can.

It's very easy for your imagination to run wild. You'll probably keep thinking about all the things that can possibly go wrong. You'll worry about every symptom. You may also have fears about how serious lupus can be, and how it can affect you and the people close to you. So learn the facts about your condition. This is a great way to alleviate some of the anxiety caused by the diagnosis. Remember, everyone is different. Some people have very mild cases of lupus with mild symptoms, while others are more seriously affected.

The emotions stemming from the diagnosis of lupus can be unpleasant. You may engage in prolonged periods of regret, sorrow, and nostalgia, remembering the way things used to be. Many fears may come to mind, some of which can be overwhelming. Fear of incapacitation, of being handicapped, and of losing friends are all very understandable fears. Begin facing them. They can and must be faced in order for you to make your adjustment. Speaking to other people who have lupus and finding out how they've adjusted can be very helpful.

WHAT'S NEXT?

Once you have become more familiar with your condition and understand how it affects you, what can you do to deal with it? For one thing, you can find out what specific changes may have to be made in your lifestyle. There is no way of knowing how many changes you'll have to make to create the best possible life for yourself.

Obviously, you should work with a physician you can trust—one who has had experience working with people having lupus before. It's usually recommended that people with lupus be treated by a board-certified rheumatologist.

You have the right to learn as much as possible about all the available treatments. How can you find out about them? Start by asking questions of your physician. Remember, the patient-physician relationship is very important in lupus. If your physician does not seem receptive to your questions, then you may have to reconsider seeing him or her. Because a chronic illness is ongoing, the patient-physician relationship will be ongoing as well. You will have much more contact with your physician because of your lupus. Some say this relationship is like a marriage, but unfortunately, you're not entitled to 50 percent of your doctor's assets if you separate!

How About the Family?

A very important part of your adjustment to a diagnosis of lupus is your family's ability to learn to adjust as well. It's hard for everyone if those around you have difficulty accepting your condition. Dealing with the diagnosis can be hard for family members. They, too, will go through periods of denial when they will say, "No, everything will be fine" or "I'm sure the problem will clear up by itself."

Ann Marie, a 34-year-old nurse, had only recently been diagnosed as having lupus. After a few depressing weeks, however, she began to learn how to cope. She was finally able to handle thoughts of lifestyle changes, concerns about reduced mobility, and some of the other unpleasant thoughts associated with lupus. Sound great? Not really. You see, her husband of fourteen years couldn't admit she had a problem, her children were afraid that she was going to die, and even her 68-year-old mother was considering selling her ranch in Texas to move closer. Although Ann Marie was learning how to cope with lupus, she could not cope with her family. They couldn't handle it, and were making things very difficult for her.

It's a great idea for family members to seek out people that they can speak to about lupus. They, too, can find out more about lupus and about how others cope with treatment. Family members can follow the same suggestions given for the person with lupus: seeking self-help groups, speaking to physicians, and reading. So encourage family members and any willing friends to learn as much as they can. This will help your adjustment.

IN A NUTSHELL

Start thinking positively about your life with lupus. Learn as much as you can about your condition. Use whatever support systems are necessary to help you. Use all the stress management and emotional control procedures available. Start saying to yourself, "Lupus may be affecting me, but I'm still alive and I'm going to do whatever I can to help myself adjust to this." If it's necessary for you to make changes in your lifestyle, even major ones, tell yourself that you will make them, and that you will make them willingly! You are going to lead as complete a life as you can. The more quickly you can adjust your lifestyle to fit your needs, the more rapidly you will be able to enjoy your life. These changes may be hard for you to adjust to at first and will take time. But at least you can be grateful that you are not helpless and can take steps to make the most of your life with lupus!

6

Depression

Jackie was depressed. A 33-year-old mother of two, married for six years and living in a comfortable home in a good neighborhood, she apparently had everything she could ask for—and lupus. She didn't ask for that. She found herself feeling increasingly upset with the changes that had to be made in her life. She felt that she could never make plans to do something and that she could never see her friends. She couldn't spend time with her children. She felt both helpless and hopeless. Jackie was suffering from depression.

Depression is a serious problem. The very mention of the word can sometimes knock the smile right off your face. Actual numbers vary, but it is estimated that more than 2 million Americans need professional care for depression. Because it is so widespread, depression has been nicknamed the "common cold" of emotional problems.

Just what is depression? Depression is an extremely unpleasant feeling of unhappiness and despair. It can range from mild, where you may feel discouraged and downhearted, to severe, where you can feel utterly hopeless, worthless, and unwilling to go on living. You may feel that there is no reason to remain a part of this world.

Depression can be painful. Imagine how it must hurt to feel or say, "I wish I were never born. What good am I? I'm not helping anybody around me and I'm not helping myself." It may seem as if life and the world are against you. Life may seem unfair—a constant struggle in which you never win. That hurts.

DEPRESSION AFFECTS YOUR BODY

The more noticeable symptoms of depression may be physical. Nervous activity or agitation, such as wringing of the hands, may occur. You may be restless, or have difficulty remaining in one place. On the other hand, you may become much less active, and remain motionless for abnormally long periods of time, appearing as if you are almost in a trance, with no apparent desire to do anything. Jim became very concerned when his 28-year-old wife, Jane, remained seated in a chair in the living room for hours at a time. When he asked her a question, she would respond in monosyllables. When friends called on the phone, she never wanted to talk to them. Jane's depression was causing her to lose interest in just about everything.

Other physical changes that can occur if you're depressed are a reduction or increase in appetite, a decreased interest in sex, and, for some women, a cessation of menstruation. If you're mildly depressed, you may have difficulty concentrating, and your attention span may be much shorter. Guys may remain unshaven simply because they don't feel like shaving. When you speak, and you'll probably do less of that, too, your conversation is more likely to be shallow, emphasizing your feelings of worthlessness and despair. Most of your physical activities will also slow down, not just because of lupus restrictions, but because of your depression.

You'll probably feel exhausted. This may seem surprising, since you're not doing much of anything anyway. But constantly telling yourself that you're no good can be very tiring! You really don't want to believe this, but you feel like you have no choice. In attempting to escape these feelings, you may become even more depressed, as well as more physically drained and exhausted.

Depression may cause you to feel physically sick. This is one of the many ways your body reacts when you're depressed. Any of the depressive symptoms we've talked about thus far might be related to a physical disorder. But if the symptoms go away when your depression improves, don't just assume that they're related to the depression. A medical examination may still be a good idea. This way, you'll be sure that there is no organic disease causing your depression.

DEPRESSION AFFECTS YOUR MOOD

You may experience frequent mood swings. For example, you might feel worse in the morning and better in the evening. This may be because of joint stiffness and pain, as well as depression. Another reason you may feel better in the evening is that you realize it's almost time to go to sleep—a means of escape. But depression may also cause difficulty sleeping, even if you weren't doing much of anything during the day.

When you're depressed, you feel like your mood keeps getting "lower." You like yourself very little, if at all. Your thinking is very negative—very different from the way it is when you're feeling good.

It is your negative thinking, not just a particular triggering event, that leads to your depression. This negative thinking tends to be the most frequently overlooked and misunderstood part of depression. Recognizing this is an important first step to learning to cope with depression.

DEPRESSION AFFECTS RELATIONSHIPS WITH OTHERS

If you're depressed, you may feel that people around you have no need for you. You may feel the same way Jackie did. She used to complain, "Why should my friends want to see me or make plans with me? They know that I'm probably going to have to change my plans. Even if I don't cancel my plans, they probably think I'll be so tired that I won't be much fun to be with anyway, so why should they even want me as a friend?" It doesn't matter how they behave toward you, you're convinced they are doing so out of obligation or necessity. You may feel that others consider you to be an uninteresting, boring person.

Do you feel less at ease talking to others? Does it seem as if others are having a hard time talking to you, even if they have been close to you for a long time? Because of your depression, you may be less interested in conversation, and less confident. You may project your feelings of self-worthlessness onto others, believing that they really don't want to talk to you. The more depressed you are, the more persuasive you may be in convincing other people around you that you are no good.

Heather received a telephone call from her friend Ann. Ann wanted to know how Heather had been feeling, since the last time they had gotten together, Heather had seemed to be in a great deal of pain. Heather responded half-heartedly, sensing that Ann was calling only out of obligation. She then explained that she would understand if Ann did not want to call again, since she never seemed to have any good news to tell her. How do you think Ann felt? Imagine hearing this repeatedly, despite reassuring Heather that her concern was sincere. Would you be surprised if Ann eventually got tired of trying to convince Heather and stopped calling? In Heather's mind, this would only reinforce the fact that she really was no good, and that she was not worthy of having any friends after all!

DEPRESSION AFFECTS PHYSICAL ACTIVITIES

Do you find that you are getting less satisfaction from your normal activities? Are you functioning like a robot? Does it seem like something is missing? It can be depressing to realize that something you used to enjoy no longer gives you the same pleasure, especially if you don't know why. It almost seems as if there is a force propelling you to "go through the motions," while your heart just isn't in it. It is understandable, therefore, that if you are depressed, you might prefer to withdraw from such activities.

WHAT CAUSES DEPRESSION?

A bout of depression frequently seems to start with one specific thing, an event or occurrence that makes you unhappy. Gloria had been planning a big dinner party for over two months. Although she had been more tired recently, she still was able to go with a friend to buy a beautiful cocktail dress. In the weeks prior to the party, she tried to get as much rest as possible. The big day finally came. Gloria felt so physically weak that she had to talk herself into getting through it. She tried to think about seeing her friends and relatives, the money she had spent on her dress, and the feeling that she did not want to give in to her lupus. But what happened? She had no choice but to sit the entire evening because she was too weak to get up. When the party was over, she was so depressed and weak that she remained in bed, crying and miserable, for over a week. That one evening triggered a long depression. She felt as if even the most important things to her were ruined because of lupus.

What happens after that first depressing event occurs? A kind of chain reaction follows. This one occurrence creates feelings that spread like wildfire. It's almost as if the bottom has dropped out of your world. You may feel less able to control your thinking (although this is not true, as we will see later). But keep in mind: The deeper you go into depression, the harder it is to climb back out again. Therefore, you certainly want to catch these feelings of depression as early as possible to try to keep yourself from spiraling further downward.

Why do we experience depression? Sometimes we can figure this out, and sometimes we can't. But before we give up, let's discuss some of the possible causes.

How About the Normal "Downs"?

A certain amount of depression is normal in anyone's life. Nobody's life is a constant "upper." We all normally experience cycles of ups and downs. If we never experienced some of the downs, how could we ever fully appreciate the ups? However, when depression becomes more than just the "normal downs," then it must be attended to. Nipping it quickly in the bud can keep it from becoming much worse.

There are certain things in anyone's life that can understandably lead to depression. Traumatic experiences such as losing a loved one, being diagnosed with a chronic illness, requiring major surgery, and being fired from a job can certainly lead to depression. That would be understandable. However, this doesn't mean you should ignore the problem or wait until it goes away. It's essential to learn how to deal with depression, since this is so important in learning how to cope with lupus.

How About Anger You Can't Express?

What if you get so angry that you feel as if you're going to burst? But you don't (or can't) do anything about it, so you decide to "swallow" it. It seems strange that a powerful feeling like anger can turn into a withdrawn, helpless feeling like depression. But it's true. If you become increasingly angry about something and feel unable to do anything about it, you may turn the anger inward. You may feel so much frustration or hopelessness that you "shut down" in an attempt to keep yourself from these terrible feelings. This leads to withdrawal, which is a symptom of depression.

Is It All in Our Minds?

A small percentage of depression cases may be caused by biochemical deficiencies—some chemical imbalance in our bodies—however, this does not occur very often. Treatment for biochemical deficiencies may involve the administration of drugs in an effort to rebalance the chemicals in our bodies. Taking medication usually isn't the whole answer. But regardless of whether your depression is caused by this or, more typically, by your reactions to things, people, and events, you should still try to modify your behavior and improve your thinking. Many experts believe that even if the cause of depression is biochemical, working on improving your thoughts and behaviors can have a positive effect on your depression.

How About Lupus?

Can lupus cause depression? Are you kidding? Living with lupus can certainly create depression or magnify already existing depression.

The depression you felt after being diagnosed with lupus is understandable. But it can get better as you begin to adjust to your new life situation. There's a problem, though. Because life with lupus has its ups and downs (physically), your feelings may bounce up and down as well. This can be a problem, considering what depression can do to you. Unfortunately, it can take a fairly long period of time (an average of two years) to adjust to having lupus. So, if your depression lingers, don't wait until you've fully adjusted to having lupus before you start learning how to cope with depression.

You may be saying to yourself, "If I'm depressed over my lupus, how can I expect to get over my depression unless I get rid of this disease?" That kind of thinking will get you nowhere. Even if you go into remission, you still can't ignore the fact that your lupus is a chronic condition. So if your depression lingers, don't wait. Work on it. Learn how to cope with it. We'll discuss how you can improve your thinking later in this chapter.

What else about lupus might depress you? You might become depressed thinking about the future, not knowing what your prognosis is or how it will affect your life. Knowing that you'll probably need medication to keep your condition from getting worse can be depressing. You might get depressed if you read misleading information in books or magazines, hear things from others ("Gee, that's a bad illness, isn't it?"), or realize how little is known about the illness. Changes in habits necessitated by your condition and its treatment may also be depressing.

The way your body feels or looks also may depress you. Experiencing a lot of pain, especially for prolonged periods of time, can be depressing. You might get depressed because you have to take medications, regardless of whether you're concerned about their side effects, the damage to your body, or the way they change your appearance.

Problems involving other people may depress you. You may feel helpless at not being able to share what you're experiencing or the way you feel. You may get depressed if others don't understand what you're going through (not that you want to be pitied, though!). People may expect more from you than you're able to (or want to) provide. They may lose confidence in you, feeling you're less reliable because of the effects of lupus. You may be depressed over the possibility of damaged relationships, lost friendships, or family friction. If you're single, you may become depressed because you think you'll never meet anyone or be able to develop a meaningful relationship because of the changes in your life necessitated by lupus.

Depression can result from changes in lifestyle. You might not be able to participate in activities you used to enjoy. You might have to change your work routine as well as your family routine. Money problems, with no immediate solution imminent, can certainly be depressing. Just having lupus, with its intangible effects on your day-to-day living, can get to you.

WHAT MAINTAINS DEPRESSION?

You may be blaming yourself or your lupus for everything that is wrong. You may tend to become more and more withdrawn, and pull away from the world around you. Why? Well, if you believe that your condition is causing all these horrible things, isn't it better to "escape" and not think about it? Realistically, escaping doesn't solve anything. But if you're depressed, you may feel that withdrawal is the only way to solve your dilemma; however, it will only keep you depressed or may, in fact, make you even more depressed.

Although you may seem sullen and withdrawn to others, you're probably in deep emotional pain. Part of what makes and keeps you depressed is your failure to protect yourself from this emotional pain. When your mind does allow any thoughts to enter, you tend to feel overwhelmed by feelings of doom and destruction. You feel that nothing good can possibly happen—that only bad things can happen. So what do you do? You try to block everything out of your mind!

So why do you stay depressed? Why doesn't the depression just go away? Perhaps because you don't want to talk to anybody, or won't even consider therapy. Therefore, the thoughts and feelings leading to your depression tend to be kept hidden. You may ask, "Is my unwillingness to talk the only reason why I'm still depressed? If I start talking more, will that get me out of my depression?" Not necessarily. But it can be helpful to talk out your feelings. It would probably be helpful (even though you may not be too thrilled) if a close friend or family member took the initiative and engaged you in some kind of conversation (therapeutic or otherwise) or at least coerced you into doing something physical.

HOW DO WE DEAL WITH DEPRESSION?

Can anything be done to combat depression? Of course! Would I abandon you without any suggestions? First, tell yourself that the *main* reason why you're still depressed is that you have not yet taken the proper steps toward feeling better! These steps can "bring you out of the rut" and reacquaint you with the more positive, pleasant aspects of living that you'd like to experience. Don't think it's easy, though. Unfortunately, once you've fallen into depression, it takes effort, hard work, and a certain amount of persistence to pull yourself back up. The fight, however, is surely worth it. Of course, the fight can be made easier if you know of specific techniques and activities that will help.

Once you feel better, you're not going to ever want to feel that depressed again, right? Well, the strategies and techniques that are most effective in dealing with depression can also be effective in preventing you from becoming depressed again! This doesn't mean you'll never feel depressed again. It may happen. Anticipate it, so that if it does recur, you won't completely fall apart. And if it does happen, won't it be good to know that you can fight it? You *can* do something to help yourself!

Depression Treatment

Now that you're ready to fight your depression, consider the two major ways of dealing with it: being more active (in other words, *doing* something) and working on your thinking.

It can be very helpful to make a list of all the things that are depressing you. You may feel there'll be at least fifty items! But in actuality, you'll probably start running dry after six or seven. Then divide this list into two more lists: first, the things that you can do something about, and second, the things you can't do anything about. (Sound familiar? You read about this earlier in the chapter. But it really works for a number of different problems. Get physical (do something) about those items in the first list, and get thoughtful (work on your thinking) regarding those items in the second list.

Let's Get Physical

Unknowingly, you may be using a lot of energy to keep yourself depressed. You may be working hard to keep that anger inside, even if it appears to others that you are withdrawing. If your depression is anger turned within, then we can logically assume that by releasing it, feelings of depression can be eliminated. But how can you effectively release those feelings? You must find an object toward which your anger can be expressed. This may be difficult. However, it's important to release the trapped anger so that it doesn't build up further and deepen the depression.

Have you ever been in the following situation? You're sitting somewhere, depressed and withdrawn. Somebody makes an innocent remark, and you practically snap the person's head off! What happened? Whatever was said triggered the release of the internalized anger that was making you depressed. Look out, world!

Consider for a moment all the energy that is keeping you depressed. You've read about why it is important to release this energy. What kinds of activities can be helpful for this? Many types of intense physical activity can release this energy. But although being active may improve your depression, it's your thoughts that make you depressed. Physical activity can provide a great distraction, which can help you look more objectively at what's going on. That will help. But it may not teach you what you need the most: ways of fighting inappropriate thinking. Besides, lupus may not even allow you to participate in intense physical activity! Fortunately, this isn't the only way to lift depression.

Let's Get Thoughtful

So if you can "think" yourself into depression, you can obviously "think" yourself out of it. How? Your thoughts are the way in which you "talk to yourself." In fact, when it comes to talking to yourself, you're probably the biggest chatterbox you know! But if you're depressed, you're just talking yourself down. All your comments, or at least most of them, are probably put-downs—harsh statements offering little to be happy about. These can make you feel even worse. You want your inner voice to help you, not hurt you. Let's see how you can do that.

Distinguishing Fact From Fiction

Don't get defensive when I tell you that when you're depressed, you tend to distort reality. Clinical research with depressed patients has proven this. Recognize, therefore, that your thoughts are not necessarily based on what is really going on, but on your own distorted views. This is called cognitive distortion.

Is that bad? You bet your happiness it is. "Cognitive" refers to your thinking. "Distortion" means you're twisting things around and, in general, losing sight of what's real. We all tend to do this from time to time. But when you're depressed, you do it a lot, if not all the time, and it *keeps* you depressed. So how do you stop? First, you must become reacquainted with what is really happening, and with the facts. But how can you do that if you keep distorting reality? Right now, you're better off accepting somebody else's perceptions of the situation, because that person is probably a lot more objective and accurate. Since so many feelings of worthlessness are based on distorted facts, depression can be reduced, if not eliminated, once these facts are straightened out.

Angela kept moaning because none of her friends were calling her. "They don't call as much as they used to. I guess they just don't care." Her sister, Stephanie, asked her to estimate how often her friends used to call. When Angela compared this number to the current number of calls she was receiving, she realized that the numbers were almost the same. She then realized that she was probably just more sensitive because of all the changes going on in her life! Although she did not feel 100 percent better, it was good to know that she wasn't being abandoned.

Making Molehills out of Mountains

Does this imply that if you're depressed you have no real problems? Is it "all in your head"? No. Everyone has problems. If you feel good, you can handle them, but if you're depressed, you may feel overwhelmed. Each and every part of your life, regardless of how trivial or slight it may be, tends to depress you. As the depression lifts, you will again be able to deal with all of life's problems, big and small.

Self-Fulfilling Prophecy

We've discussed several different ways that you may feel if you're depressed. Are all these feelings irrational and untrue? No. Ironically, although some of them may start off being far from the truth, the longer you feel that way, the more chance there will be for your feelings to become "self-fulfilling prophecies." In other words, you'll begin convincing yourself that nonsense makes sense. For example, if you begin telling yourself that friends and relatives don't care, this may become a reality because your negative attitude may alienate the people close to you. They may decide you're not worth the bother. As far as your activities go, you are less likely to do anything when you're depressed. You'll probably be less likely to even attempt doing the things you used to enjoy. As a result, you'll feel less competent and will not accomplish anything. This will tend to magnify and confirm your feelings of worthlessness, leading to even greater depression. Not a pretty picture.

Once you begin feeling depressed, your negative thoughts will soon lead to negative actions. These negative actions will lead to more negative thoughts, which will in turn lead to more negative actions, and so on. It is an ongoing, vicious circle that will spiral you further downward into deeper depression. Eventually, you'll feel trapped in this vicious circle with no way to escape from the "dumps."

Are you getting depressed just reading this? In all probability, if you've ever been depressed, you've said to yourself at least once already, "Wow, that sounds just like me!" So you see, your negative thoughts become self-fulfilling prophecies. If you find that you are starting to believe in your negative thoughts, stop yourself. Try to think positive thoughts, so that if your thoughts *do* turn out to be real, they will at least be positive ones.

Positive Is the Opposite of Negative

As we've said before, depression results from and causes a lot of negative thinking. Negative thoughts automatically pop into your mind and you cannot stop them. It's like trying to keep your eyes open when you sneeze! You just can't do it. But once you become aware of them, then you can do something. People who remain depressed feel incapable of doing anything about their negative thinking, and allow these thoughts to continue. They simply continue in that vicious, downward circle that was mentioned earlier.

Ann, a 34-year-old housewife, was resting when the telephone rang. "I'm sure that's Katherine, calling to cancel our lunch plans," she thought to herself. Within the thirty seconds it took her to get to the phone, she had become so depressed that she considered not even answering the call. Imagine how she felt when she reluctantly answered the phone and discovered that it was a wrong number! Ann had allowed her negative thoughts to run wild—she became more and more negative until she was about ready to give up. And for what? There was no clear-cut reason for thinking the way she did.

Once she realized that she was thinking this way, what could she have done? She could have countered her thoughts. She could have told herself, "It may not even be Katherine on the phone. Or if it is, maybe she's just calling to confirm. I won't let it bother me now. After all, I don't even know who it is." This is the beginning of positive thinking.

Dwell on the Brighter Tomorrows

Marie was depressed because she constantly compared her present condition to the way she used to be. She couldn't swim anymore, stay out late with the girls, spend hours in museums, or participate in many other of her favorite activities. She allowed these thoughts to overwhelm her, and, as a result, certainly did not give herself a chance to enjoy her life.

If you find yourself unhappily comparing your present life to life before lupus, try to modify your thinking. Start planning fun things for the present and future. Anyone can come up with some enjoyable things to do, regardless of how restricted the person may be. But it takes effort. Don't wallow in self-pity; it will only allow your depression to strangle you. Work on your thinking, develop some positive plans, and translate them into pleasure. Then wave good-bye to your depression!

When you recall the past, you may not even think it was that much better. You may have had other physical problems. You may have made some mistakes in your life. This may make you even more depressed about the future. However, you can't change the past. What's done is done. Keep telling yourself that. Tell yourself that you're going to work on making the future better. Set up some specific goals, starting with the easy-to-reach ones. You'll be helping yourself just by thinking about what you can do that's more positive. Don't punish yourself for the past.

What's Missing From Your Life?

You may have laughed when you read the heading to this section. "Good health," you might respond. "Mobility without pain!" Sure. But why discuss this? Because depressed people frequently lament the fact that something is missing from their lives. What is usually missing is a feeling of satisfaction, accomplishment, and pride that normally comes from others' praise. You may just miss the attention and interest of other people. This may cause you to feel worthless. How do you counteract this? Think about your positive qualities (yes, you do have some!). Think about how you can interact with people more, spark their interest, and become more satisfied with yourself.

Shoot for the Earth, Not the Moon

We all have goals for ourselves. It's normal to become depressed when we don't reach a particular goal, especially if we've tried very hard to get there. But maybe the goal you set is not a realistic one. Maybe you're trying to do something you can't, and you're getting depressed instead of realistically resetting your goal.

Jenny had not returned to work since a major flare had required a six-week stay in the hospital. Finally, after a long period of rest and medication, she was feeling better and was looking forward to getting back to work so she could catch up on everything. When her doctor finally gave her the "go ahead," she practically flew to her office. After two hours of phone calls, typing, dictation, and meetings, she was exhausted. Her spirits plummeted. She became worried that she wouldn't be able to handle all the pressure, and that she was in danger of losing her job. Wrong! Jenny had simply set her sights too high. Expecting to return to her old schedule as if she didn't have lupus was just not realistic. Try to return to your old activities slowly. Build up your stamina. Isn't the end result more important than the initial gains? And if your goals are more realistically set, you'll have a much better chance of achieving them, and less of a chance of falling short.

AN ANTIDEPRESSING SUMMARY

The best way to work on negative thoughts is to prevent them from continuing. Try to be more positive, and make realistic goals for yourself. Deal with reality the way it actually exists. Deal with thoughts from a more factual point of view. Deal with them the way somebody else might—somebody who is not depressed and who can be more objective. Try to make your perceptions more accurate, your awareness more realistic, and your thoughts more positive and constructive. Remember: Your thoughts lead to your emotions. If your thoughts are negative and critical, then your emotions will also be in bad shape. If you can turn your thoughts around to a more positive, constructive point of view, you'll see that your emotional reactions will improve as well.

7

Fears and Anxieties

Don't be "afraid" to read this chapter! It may help you discover what you're "anxious" about!

The two sentences above may help you distinguish between fear and anxiety. What's the difference? *Anxiety* is a general sense of uneasiness—a vague feeling of discomfort. It is an agitated, uncertain state in which you just don't feel at peace or in control. There is a premonition that something bad may happen which you have to protect yourself against. You feel very vulnerable. However, you're not exactly sure what the source of your anxiety is.

Fear, on the other hand, is usually more specific. It's often directed toward something that can be recognized, whether it's a person, object, situation, or event. We experience fear when we become aware of something dangerous, or when we feel threatened. When we are afraid (as with feeling anxious), we also feel out of control and less confident. So the feelings of fear and anxiety are basically the same. The main difference is whether you can identify the source of the feeling. From this point on, however, I'll be using the two terms interchangeably so that there is less confusion.

Fear is so prevalent that many words are used to describe it: scared, concerned, alarmed, worried, uptight, nervous, edgy, shaky. Then there's perplexed, wary, frightened, helpless, frustrated. Is that it? Nope! How about suspicious, keyed-up, impatient, giddy, hesitant, apprehensive, tense, panicky, disturbed, agitated? Of course, there are more, but if I went on this book would have to be renamed *The Fear Synonym Book*. All these words mean the same thing: "I'm afraid." The source of this fear may be real or imaginary.

IS FEAR GOOD OR BAD?

Believe it or not, fear is usually good! Now you're probably saying, "If I'm shaking with fear, how can it be good?" For one thing, fear mobilizes you. It "tells" you to prepare to attack the source of your fear. You react in a way that leads to action. In this regard, fear is similar to stress. It serves a necessary and critical purpose. In a way, it "protects" you.

Fear is bad only if it is denied, or if it is so excessive that you can't do anything about it. If you face your fear and push past it, trying to resolve it, then fear is a positive emotion. It is only when the source ·of fear becomes overlooked, ignored, or denied that the consequences may be a problem, because the threat or danger is allowed to continue, and nothing or not enough is being done to control it.

HOW INTENSE ARE OUR REACTIONS?

Fear ranges in intensity from mild to severe. It is impossible to measure how much fear there is in anyone's life. It is unique and varies from person to person.

What determines how fearful you get? Usually the strength of the feared object, person, or event is important. Also important is how close it is (wouldn't you be more afraid of getting an injection within the next thirty seconds than if you were getting it in thirty days?); how vulnerable you are (do you hate injections, or are you just tired of feeling like a pincushion?); and how successful you are in conducting yourself (can you calmly accept the needle, or do you scream a lot?). These are some of the factors determining how you handle fear. Your own strength and the success of your defense mechanisms also play a role.

Becky, aged 29, was afraid to go to sleep at night. She was worried that she'd wake up in the morning with painful lupus symptoms. Since she felt fine at night, she didn't want to go to sleep. If Becky was stronger (emotionally), she might still be concerned about new symptoms, but would not let them disturb her sleep. Becky, however, wasn't strong; she was frightened. Her fear kept her awake, she got less sleep, and she became more vulnerable to the very symptoms she wanted to avoid!

People with lupus can be afraid of many things. Obviously, the more fears you have, the more they can interfere with your successful adjustment. Recognizing your fears and learning how to deal with them will help you live more happily and more comfortably. How? I was afraid you'd never ask!

HOW TO COPE WITH FEARS AND ANXIETIES

The first step in coping with your fears is to use the "pinpointing" technique discussed in Chapter 4. List all the things you're afraid of. Identify exactly what you are afraid of and exactly why you are afraid. Then think about what you can do to alleviate your fears.

For Claudia, this was not hard. She knew she was afraid of how people would react when they saw the rash on her face. She quickly realized that what she feared was rejection. She was concerned that they wouldn't want to be with her because of their own fears ("Is it contagious?" "Will it affect me?" "I don't want to be seen with her," and so on). She planned a course of action (no, not a one-way ticket to Brazil!). She decided she'd simply do the best she could, expecting her friends to accept her the way she was. If they didn't, that was *their* loss. She was less afraid almost instantly. As you begin planning your strategies and gradually put your plan into operation, you'll continue to feel better and better.

Desensitize Yourself

A great technique used to conquer fear is called systematic desensitization. You learn to desensitize yourself to make yourself less vulnerable to the source of your fear.

Here's how to try it. Sit in a comfortable chair and relax. Then create a movie in your mind. Imagine what it is that makes you afraid. If you get tense, stop imagining it and relax. When you've calmed down, try imagining it again. The more you try to imagine your fear, the less it will bother you. Try it! It will give you a great feeling of relaxation and control. There are several library books that provide more information on systematic desensitization. Check them out.

It was stated earlier that anxiety is a vague, uneasy feeling with an unknown source. So how can you cope with it by following the steps listed above? Well, if you try to pinpoint the source and are unable to, then you probably can't follow the steps. So what can you do? Use relaxation procedures. Work on changing your thinking. Even if you can't pinpoint a specific fear, these techniques will greatly help you to cope with general anxiety.

LET'S TALK ABOUT SPECIFICS

Remember, it is understandable for you to have many fears related to your condition. A problem, however, arises when you don't admit these fears. As a result, you don't do anything about resolving them. They can be resolved. And you can work on changing your thinking.

Initial Fears

When you were first diagnosed, many fearful questions probably came to mind. "What will the future be like? What will become of me? Will I die?" These are all legitimate questions and justifiable fears. But time goes on. Some of these questions have been answered, and some of your initial qualms about having lupus have not materialized. But you're probably still afraid of some things. Let's discuss some of them.

Fear of Dying

Although the mortality rate for lupus has been greatly reduced, it still has not been eliminated, so being afraid of dying is understandable. When might you be most afraid of dying? Probably when you're in the middle of a flare, or when your symptoms are particularly rough. Beginning a new treatment or being involved in any of the ups and downs that remind you of your vulnerability can also cause these fears. When you feel the worst, you're more likely to fear the worst. However, being afraid of dying is not going to help you feel better or live longer. If anything, it's only going to make you feel worse! Being afraid of dying, therefore, falls into the category of fears that you can do little or nothing about. How do you attack this fear? Research is constantly exploring new and improved treatment possibilities for individuals with lupus. So think positively. Others have had worse symptoms and still live comfortably. Do you see how you must work on your thinking? If negative thoughts make you more afraid, then positive thoughts . . .

When you're feeling better and have fewer symptoms, you're less likely to be afraid of dying. At that point you're more likely to be afraid of going into another flare.

Fear of a Flare

Of course, sometimes even if you're doing everything perfectly, you'll still go into a flare. Can you defeat this fear? Yes. Try to plan what you're going to do when a flare occurs. For example, if you're afraid that a flare will affect your work, plan in advance how you're going to handle your job, your employer, and your responsibilities if and when it does happen.

Fear of Pain

Nobody likes pain. Pain is one of the most unpleasant problems associated with lupus. You may be afraid of pain. This fear may be just as strong when you don't have pain, since you're afraid of it's happening! If you do feel pain, you'll wonder when you're going to feel some relief. Each little twinge of pain may make you afraid that further deterioration of your condition will occur, or that additional problems exist or may develop. What can you do about this fear? Try to accept the fact that some pain may be with you from time to time, but medication can reduce its intensity. Further suggestions will be offered in Chapter 14, "Pain." Realize that each pain cycle will eventually stop or at least ease up. It won't last forever.

Fear of Medication and Possible Side Effects

You may be nervous about the different medications that you have to take, even though you need them. You may be afraid of what they're doing to your body. Just keep reminding yourself about the damage lupus could do to you without medication! Your physician is aware of the possible side effects, but will still prescribe medication as long as the advantages of the medication outweigh the side effects, and the side effects are not as potentially dangerous as uncontrolled lupus.

What if you've had problems with your treatment? What if all the therapies you've tried haven't seemed to have done any good? If it seems as if you experience unpleasant side effects with every medication you try, you may begin to fear that nothing is going to work. Unfortunately, there are some people who have more difficulty than others finding the right "formula." And it's possible you may not benefit as much as you (and your doctor, family, therapists, and friends, and others) would like. But hang in there. New medications and techniques are being developed all the time. And, who knows? More trial and error may result in a solution. Giving up will just make you more tense and uncomfortable anyway. So keep trying.

Fear of What Will Happen Next

What will happen next? You can't be sure. Will there be an increase in the amount of pain? Will you develop new symptoms? Will you develop new side effects from your medication? Will you go into or stay in remission? When will you have another flare? Fear of the future course of the illness includes being afraid of new symptoms, or the return of old ones.

Everyone wonders what's in store for the future. But because of the unpleasantness of what you've experienced, you may be afraid of the future, rather than merely curious. What can you do? Unless you own a crystal ball, you can't foresee what will happen in the future. So take life one day at a time. What will be, will be. (What a great name for a song!) Just tell yourself that you'll handle any problems as they occur.

Fear of Not Being Believed

Are you in pain? Do you find it hard to let other people know about your pain? Maybe you're afraid that they won't believe you. "I can't believe that anybody would experience as many symptoms and as much pain as you do with lupus," you're afraid they're thinking. How can you have energy and be able to function one minute, and the very next minute be so tired that you can barely move out of the chair? It may seem strange, but you know it's true; however, it's frightening to think that other people just will not understand. You don't want to be labelled a hypochondriac! Talk to the nonbelievers. Share reading material with them. Try to explain lupus as best as you can. You've then done all you can. You can't crawl into someone else's head and change his or her beliefs.

Fear of Disability

The thought of being disabled may be horrible. Because you know that lupus can cause severe physical restrictions in some cases, you may have this fear. But being "disabled" is a bad term, since it suggests that you can't do anything. If you look around you and think more objectively, you'll realize that a physical disability wouldn't make you any less of a human being. You would still have many, many capabilities. Numerous Olympic champions began their athletic careers to overcome physical disabilities. Beethoven wrote some of his greatest music after becoming totally deaf. There was even a one-armed baseball player in the major leagues. Regardless of their disabilities, these people all had one thing in common: the knowledge that they could overcome or at least compensate for a limitation in one area by developing abilities in another.

How might a disability affect you? You might have a tendency to become increasingly dependent on others, since you can't do as much for yourself. You may be afraid that you'll lose your ability to get around because of joint pain or arthriticlike symptoms. Once again, it's your thinking that's making you afraid. Other than trying to take good care of yourself, what else can you really do? Take things as they come, but think more positively. Remember: You still have lots of room for self-fulfillment.

If you are already disabled, this can certainly be frightening, especially if you enjoy independence. You don't want to be a burden to the important people in your life. Can you do anything about this? That depends on the nature of your disability. Find out everything you can about the possibility of rehabilitation. If there's any chance, take advantage of it. Even if there's no possibility of total rehabilitation, every little bit helps. Just don't let yourself collapse, or you'll be doing yourself an enormous disservice.

Fear of the Reactions of Others

Are you afraid that other people will not accept you with lupus? Do you fear they may shun you for physical reasons? You may fear rejection if you can't socialize the way you'd like to be able to. Others may feel that you can't keep up with them. But don't try to, because pushing yourself can be a painful way to maintain a friendship.

Unfortunately, some people can be cold and unfeeling and may have trouble dealing with you the way you are. Who needs those kinds of friends anyway? Other friends will accept you under any circumstances. Enjoy them. But since you can't change the way some people feel, try not to be as concerned with their reactions. Instead, be more attentive to your own needs and feelings.

Other fears in this category can be even more frightening. "What if my spouse leaves me? What if all my friends stay away from me?" Fear of desertion can be horrible. If it's not happening now, you may be afraid of it happening in the future. You may be afraid that none of your friends will remain "in your corner." To reduce the chances of such rejection, you may hesitate to make plans with friends or family. This will only add to your feeling of isolation.

Consider your thoughts, but be realistic. Remember that a change in a social relationship can occur for any reason, not just because of lupus. If you feel that a relationship is in jeopardy, see what you can do to help—"put all your cards on the table," discuss any problems, and even get counseling if you need it. But you can do only so much. If that doesn't work, even though the outcome may upset you, at least you'll know you've tried.

Fear of Overdoing/Undergoing

You may not know how much you should do. You may be afraid of doing too much, but you may feel guilty about doing too little! How do you conquer this? Get advice from experts. You need professional advice in order to come up with the best mix of rest and exercise. This may become apparent only through trial and error. You can learn only through experience. Pace yourself. Change your level of activity gradually. Then tell yourself, as with so many other fears, that you're doing the best you can.

Fear of Going Out

Are you afraid to go out? You may think you're going to get tired or get sick. Maybe you're concerned about collapsing from weakness and not being helped. Jeannie planned a very pleasant outing to the city only to find that very shortly after she got there, she was no longer able to walk around! Are you afraid you'll get so tired that it will take hours to complete a simple chore? You may also be afraid of getting sick while you're out. You may be concerned about getting the help you would need if you fainted or couldn't move. You may also be concerned about how others will look at you or treat you. It is understandable to feel afraid of these things, but does that justify your staying home all the time? That won't help you get over these fears. There are some things you *can* do to reduce your fears. If you plan ahead, you will feel more at ease. If you're concerned about your physical state, take someone with you when you go out instead of going alone. Pace yourself. Plan your activities for times when you're the most rested, and don't try to do too much at once.

Fear of Traveling

If you worry about going out, you may also be reluctant to travel with lupus. Why? You wouldn't know the doctors, what kind of medical facilities would be available, or who you could contact if you experienced a problem. You also don't even know if lupus is understood by the medical professionals of that country, and you certainly don't want to have to explain! Obviously, if you travel by car, this may not be as much of a problem. You're not going to be so far away that you couldn't get help if you really needed it. But you may not be sure you can walk as much as you'd like on your trip, or whether your destinations are conducive to your getting around.

What can you do? By planning in advance, you should be able to conquer your fears. Ask your doctor if he knows of any doctors or facilities where you're planning to go. You might want to contact them in advance just to be reassured that they're there, that they know about lupus, and that they know you're coming. If your physician has no contacts, try to get some names on your own (try the local medical society or your local chapter of the Lupus Foundation), or plan your vacation at a place where adequate medical services are available. Plan on not overdoing it. Visiting five landmarks in one day is a bit much! (More about this in Chapter 20, "Traveling.")

Fear of Employment Problems and Lost Income

You may be concerned about whether you'll be able to keep your job. You may want to work, but fear that you won't be able to. Your employer may be understanding at first, but you may worry about how long this will continue. Can you do anything to reduce your fears? You can evaluate your vocational skills and make sure you have a job that you can handle. Other than this, you'll have to live with this fear, and just hope for the best. If there's a problem, you'll cope with it. Being afraid won't help.

If you can't work, the financial pressure is even greater. Medical bills have to be paid. You can't depend on insurance plans, since they don't always provide enough coverage. In addition, many insurance plans require you to pay the doctor first and then get reimbursed. Doctors' fees can be quite high, and if the money is not coming in, what can you do? Talk to people. Speak to others with lupus who cannot work. Find out what they are doing to cope. Maybe you'll get some ideas that will help you conquer this fear.

Fear That Your Child Will Inherit Lupus

The thought of transmitting lupus to your children may be so frightening that you may not want to have children. But even if you already

have a family, you may be panicky. You don't want to live in constant
fear of your child saying that a joint hurts or showing you a rash on
that little face! Learn the facts. A tendency toward lupus may be genetically transmitted, but the chances are very small that your child
will develop the disease. Symptoms can occur in anyone, with or
without lupus. Just because your child has one of the symptoms of lupus, it doesn't mean that he or she has the condition. Speak to your
doctor, and relax.

If your child is diagnosed with lupus, it need not be the end of the
world. It's not your fault. Your child still "wanted" to be born and to
be alive. Maybe you'll be able to help one another adjust. But don't
resign yourself to the fact that your child is destined to get lupus until
a diagnosis is made. Otherwise, you'll be blowing your fear all out of
proportion. Remember, treatment is improving and will likely be
even better when your child is growing up than it is now. A diagnosis
of lupus need not be a disaster.

Fear of Not Coping

You may feel that you're barely handling having lupus. You may think
that any new problem that comes along will be enough to push you
over the edge. Fear of falling apart can easily lead to panic, an out-of-
control kind of feeling that will make you fall apart. Get a hold of
yourself. Pinpoint those particular things you're having difficulty
with and get help in dealing with them. Don't wait. Don't project a
false sense of bravado that you can and must handle everything yourself. If you feel yourself nearing the edge, get someone to help you to
steady yourself. Talk things over with someone. Once you share your
feelings and fears with someone, you may see things a little more
clearly. You may have greater strength to deal with your problems,
knowing that you're not alone. Once you're back in control, your
fear of not being able to cope will disappear.

A FEARLESS SUMMARY

Although many different fears have been discussed in this chapter, we
have probably not covered all of the ones you have experienced. In
addition, the coping suggestions offered certainly do not include all
possible ways of dealing with fear. So what should you do?

You're working on recognizing your fears, right? For some of
them, you're modifying your behavior. For others, you're modifying

your thinking. Soon you will feel more in control. As this happens, you'll notice your fears begin to diminish. That doesn't mean that they'll all go away. But as you work on them and feel more in control, they'll at least lessen in intensity. You'll feel better knowing that you can do something about some of them, and that you're capable of handling them.

8

Anger

It was the day of the senior prom. Linda, a 17-year-old high school student, was sitting by her telephone waiting for a call from her doctor. She had not been feeling that well, but she was hoping that the doctor would tell her that she was healthy enough to go to the prom. The telephone rang, and Linda answered. Her doctor told her the results of her blood tests; they showed that a lupus flare had begun. He said that she would be best off if she got plenty of rest, and recommended that she not go out. Barely able to say good-bye, she slammed down the telephone and threw herself on the bed, pounding on her pillow. Was Linda angry? You bet she was!

Donna, aged 31, was fed up with joint pain. Practically anyone who went near her received an earful of comments you wouldn't want your mother to hear! Everyone from her doctor to her family was a victim of this verbal assault. What made her even more angry was that she wanted to slam her fist down on her kitchen table, but she knew it would just make her pain worse. Donna was angry!

In general, any person with a restrictive physical condition may be angry. Because anger results in the build-up of physical energy that needs to be released, it is important for you to learn how to cope with anger.

WHAT IS ANGER?

When you have a desire or goal in mind, and something interferes with your fulfillment or achievement of it, a feeling of tension and hostility may result from the developing frustration. This is what we refer to as anger.

THREE TYPES OF ANGER

It can be helpful to discuss three different ways of experiencing anger. Rage is the expression of violent, uncontrolled anger. If Donna was feeling upset about her condition, and a "friend" told her that her joints would still be healthy if she had taken better care of herself, you can imagine how angry she might be. Her anger might even lead her to say or do things that would certainly not enhance the prospects of a long, warm relationship with this person! Rage is probably the most intense anger you can experience. It is an outward expression of anger, as it results in a visible explosion. Rage can be a destructive release of the intense physical energy that builds up.

A second type of anger is resentment. This is the feeling of anger that is usually kept inside. What if Donna listened to her friend's well-meaning comments, smiled, and said nothing, but was seething inside? Resentment is a growing, smoldering feeling of anger directed toward a person or an object. However, it is kept bottled up. It tends to sit uncomfortably within you, and can create even more physiological and psychological damage.

The third type of anger is indignation. Indignation is considered the more appropriate, positive type of anger. It is released in a more controlled way. Donna might have responded more appropriately to her "friend's" comments if she had stated that she appreciated her friend's concern, but would prefer no advice at this point or she might scream. Obviously, these three types of anger can occur in different ways. However, understanding the different ways of experiencing anger can help you cope with it more effectively.

CAUSES OF ANGER

Obviously, there are lots of things that can make you angry. You may get angry waiting for your doctor to see you. You wouldn't be too thrilled if you had to cancel your plans at the last moment. You may also get angry if you are told you need yet another type of medication.

Insults from other people, aside from everyday frustrations, can cause anger. "If you washed your face better, you wouldn't have those ugly splotches on your nose and cheeks." This is not the kind of comment that would make you feel friendly! If you feel that some-one is taking advantage of you or feel as if you have been forced to do something that you did not want to do, anger may result. Let's say that your friend says, "I'm going to a party next Saturday. You have such good taste in clothes, please come with me to pick out a dress. We'll go to only seven or eight stores." If you do not have the ability or confidence to say "no" when friends ask for a favor, this can cre-ate feelings of anger, especially when combined with the fact that you may not feel well.

In addition to the causes of anger mentioned above, there is one more. How about lupus as a cause of anger? Aren't you angry about having lupus? There may not be any specific reason for your anger that you can point to. Or you might be able to list dozens of reasons why lupus makes you angry. But being aware of the reasons for your anger is important, because you must be aware of them to help your-self deal with it. Unfortunately, resolving your anger won't make your lupus go away. Nor should you say that you'll stop being angry only when lupus is a thing of the past. Neither attitude will help you. As we go on, we will be discussing ways of reducing anger and feel-ing better.

Do Your Thoughts Make You Angry?

It is important to realize that anger exists uniquely in the mind of each angry individual. This anger is a direct result of your thoughts rather than events. The event by itself does not make you angry. Rather, it is your *interpretation* of the event—the way you think or feel about it—that can make you angry. This is a very important point, one that will be discussed in much more detail a little bit later in the section "Dealing With Anger." Stay tuned. . . .

EFFECTS OF ANGER ON YOUR BODY

When you are angry, a number of physiological responses occur in your body. Breathing becomes more rapid, blood pressure increases (you may feel as if your blood is "boiling"), and your heart may begin to pound. Your face may get hot, and your muscles may become tense. You may feel stronger when you are angry. The more intense your anger, the greater your feeling of power. I'm sure you can re-member a time when you were so angry that you felt you had super-human strength.

Anger is a form of energy. The more physical energy that builds up in the body due to anger, the more necessary it becomes for you to release it. The energy cannot be destroyed, so if it is not released in some constructive manner, it will eventually come out in another, less desirable way. Imagine the energy from anger as a stick of dynamite about to explode. If you get rid of it, it will explode away from you. It may cause some damage, but it will not hurt you inside as much as if you swallowed the dynamite to keep others from being hurt. Obviously, the ideal solution is not to throw the stick of dynamite and not to swallow it, but (are you ready for this?) to try to defuse the dynamite! More about defusing soon.

Usually, extreme anger can pass quickly. If, however, the anger lasts for a long period of time, it can have damaging effects on the body. You've all heard about some of the physical problems that can result from holding in anger: ulcers, hypertension, headaches. Anger can also cause a stress response that may exacerbate your lupus. It's just not good for your body.

When anger becomes extreme or turns into rage, you may feel like exploding. You may feel that unless you are able to punch, kick, or hit something or to get rid of the anger in some other way, you may lose control. Hopefully, this angry energy can be released without causing damage to another person, property, or yourself. If, when you finally calm down, you find that you have done something destructive, you may get angry at yourself all over again. Or you may experience another negative emotion, such as guilt.

EFFECTS OF ANGER ON YOUR MIND

Anger is usually experienced as an unpleasant feeling. However, this unpleasant feeling may exist along with the more pleasant feeling of power or strength. Frequently, the unpleasantness of anger is related to its consequences—knowing what you do when you are angry and not being happy about it. If you lose control when you're angry, you'll probably even be afraid of your anger, and of what you might do next time!

DIFFERENT REACTIONS TO ANGER

Maureen, a 28-year-old teacher, was having a hard time with her husband. He was trying to show concern for his wife by not letting her do any housework. But, surprisingly, she *wanted* to clean the house because she believed she felt well enough to do it. His resistance was so persistent and he was so "saccharin sweet" that Maureen felt it was too much. She wanted to be treated like an adult, able to determine when she could be active. But her husband just wouldn't let up. She was running out of patience. Let's see how Maureen might handle the situation in different ways.

The "Ignore" Approach

Because you feel as if you may completely lose control when you are angry, or feel overwhelmed by the intensity of your anger, you may try to do whatever you can to avoid the experience. This could include pushing thoughts out of your mind even when you realize you are getting angry. If Maureen uses this approach to deal with her anger, she might try to get involved in different activities while her husband cleans the house, and try to ignore the fact that he is being so condescending. Or she might try to agree with everything that he says. Although this might be upsetting to her, it might at least be temporarily effective in helping her to ignore the smothering. In the long run, however, you can see that this is not the best way to deal with anger.

The "Action" Approach

From another point of view, you might see anger as a necessary part of life, despite its unpleasantness. Whether you like it or not, there will be times when you'll be angry. You'll just have to deal with your anger as best as you can.

Because Maureen is unhappy about being angry, she might speak to her husband to try to get him to understand more about her emotional needs and about how she'd like him to treat her. Hopefully, a better understanding will be reached, but at least Maureen will know that she's doing something about her feelings.

The "Power" Approach

Maybe you enjoy the flow of energy and strength that comes from being angry. You may find that this is when you are best able to assert yourself to accomplish something. If Maureen fits this description, she might explode if she is smothered once too often by her husband.

She loves the feeling of power that her anger gives her, and is almost looking forward to the chance to say to him, "Honey, if you treat me that way once more, I'll take this vacuum cleaner and . . . !" That would wipe the smile off hubby's face!

If you enjoy this feeling, it's possible that you may even provoke situations to make yourself angry! An example of this would be professional football players or boxers who psyche themselves up before a confrontation with an opponent. For them, becoming as angry as possible is the best preparation for a successful performance.

Your own reaction to anger is unique. It may also change from time to time. There may be times when you accept anger and almost value it as a motivator to accomplish something. At other times you may attempt to push your anger away. Maureen might enjoy expressing her anger. But if she doesn't want to cause problems with or hurt her husband, or upset the rest of the family, she might realize that it would be better to have a calm discussion with him than to shatter his eardrums with her explosion.

IS ANGER GOOD OR BAD?

How can anger possibly be good? Many people feel that nothing constructive can be gained from it. "Avoid anger at all costs," they say, "because nothing good comes from it. . . . Anger will get you into trouble, so don't let it arise." This is true, but only if you don't deal with the anger properly. Anger can be dangerous if it is kept inside. Remember that stick of dynamite? What an explosive example! If anger is released in destructive ways, it can cause problems in relationships (to say the least!). It can create physical problems as well, and can certainly aggravate your lupus-related problems. Does this mean that anger can make your condition worse? Well, what if you're so angry at somebody or something that you decide not to take proper care of yourself? For example, what if you are so mad at the world that you don't take your medication properly? Taking more or less than the prescribed amount can be harmful to your health. Or what if being angry at someone or something causes you to do more than you should be doing? "I'll show them," you say. Having lupus, you know that you may eventually have to pay the price for overdoing it. What if you're angry at someone who cares about you and normally helps you deal with your lupus symptoms? That person, if upset by your anger, may be less willing to help you. This may, in turn, make you feel even worse. So if you want your anger to be good instead of bad, try to turn it into something that can be helpful rather than harmful to you.

Anger can be constructive. It can mobilize you and make you stronger to deal with an anger-provoking situation. Believe it or not, you might even handle a situation more successfully than you would if you weren't angry! Anger can give you a feeling of power or strength, of confidence or assertiveness. But don't misunderstand me. I'm not saying that you should slam your finger with a hammer or tell someone to punch you in order to get yourself angry enough to solve all of your problems! What I am saying is that anger can be positive, and it can help you to solve problems.

Anger has two main benefits. First, it is an indicator that something is wrong. Something must be creating this feeling of anger—something that needs attention. Second, anger can motivate you to deal more actively with life's problems. You can become so emotionally charged that it will have a positive effect on your life.

In order for anger to be helpful, there are some very important things to keep in mind. First, don't let yourself become overwhelmed by the anger. Once that happens, it is much harder to do what you have to do. Second, don't be afraid of your anger. If you do fear it, you probably won't be able to release it properly. More than likely, it will come out in unhealthy ways, or you'll bottle it up inside. Third, be sure that the way you handle your anger is socially acceptable. Maureen might get a kick out of knocking out her husband's teeth, but would the dentist or police approve? Try to be flexible enough to recognize an appropriate way of releasing your anger.

DEALING WITH ANGER

You've already begun to realize that anger can be constructive. Hopefully, the information you've read so far has been encouraging. But what else can actually be done to handle anger?

Because anger is such a complex emotion, and because so many things can lead to feelings of anger, there are no simple answers. Sorry about that! Does that mean that there is nothing that anybody can do about anger? No. Some things can be done to reduce feelings of anger and allow them to be handled more efficiently, comfortably, and safely.

Step One—Admit That You're Angry

The first step in dealing with anger is to recognize that you're angry in the first place. As simple as this may sound, many people cannot even admit when they are angry. They may try to deny it, or rationalize their feelings or behaviors using other explanations. Do you feel that being angry is a sign of weakness? If so, since you don't want to feel weak, you may not even admit that you're angry. You may feel that there is no appropriate reason to be angry and that you're acting in a childish way. But as with anything else, in order to try to change something, you've got to first admit that it exists.

How can you tell that you're angry if you're not sure? (Yes, there are some people who are not sure.) If you feel very tense (jumping at the sound of the telephone), or if you find yourself reacting impulsively (slamming down the phone when you get a wrong number and storming out of the house) or with hostility (cursing at your neighbor for leaving a smidgeon of garbage on your lawn), chances are that you're angry. Until you recognize that you are angry, you cannot do anything constructive about it.

Step Two—Identify What Is Making You Angry

The second step in dealing with anger is to try to identify its source. Where does it come from? What is contributing to it? What events have led to these feelings of anger? Why do you want to break all the furniture? For one thing, your condition may lead to anger. You may be angry with yourself for neglecting your condition. You may feel anger toward your physician, whether justified or not. You may be angry because you have to take so much medication. You may be angry because of the things you can no longer do.

In some cases, the events leading to anger may be quite obvious. In other cases, however, the source of anger may be vague and unclear. It may be hard to pinpoint what is causing it. At such times, you should try to probe even more deeply to come up with possible causes of your anger.

Take, for example, the case of Suzanne, a 47-year-old homemaker. She was awakened one bright, cheerful morning to hear birds singing right outside her bedroom. Instead of feeling happy and carefree, she felt angry. She had just awakened, but she felt angry. Initially, she was unable to figure out why, on such a beautiful day, she might feel angry. But finally, after giving the matter a lot of thought, she realized that because it was sunny and bright out, her detested cousins were going to come from out of town to visit, and she would feel obligated to entertain them—something that she did not wish to do. Remember: Being able to identify the source of your anger is very important in being able to deal with it.

Of course, much of this anger is irrational. But, like other emotional reactions, it must be worked through. It cannot just be pushed away. Simply telling yourself, "Don't be angry," is not enough. You must learn to channel your anger more effectively.

Guilt can sometimes confuse you if you are trying to identify the source of anger. Such was the case with Margaret, a 33-year-old mother of three. She woke up one morning, went downstairs, and found her kitchen a disaster area. Taking care of the kitchen was a responsibility that she had given to her children, because she was simply physically unable to handle it. She found herself screaming at them for not fulfilling their responsibilities. In actuality, however, her anger may have been a reflection not of hostility toward her three children, but of guilt about her own inability to handle her kitchen responsibilities.

Step Three—Identify Why You Are Angry

It is now necessary to explain to yourself why you are angry. In Margaret's case, she could explain her anger by her inability to do what she wanted to do. Margaret wanted to be able to fulfill her responsibilities as a mother and housewife. She felt that taking care of the kitchen was included in this. Because she was unable to do so, she felt angry.

Why is it important to identify why you are angry? Mainly, to decide whether the anger you are feeling is realistic. Analyze your reasons for being angry. If you recognize that your reasons are not realistic, this alone can help you deal with these feelings of anger. If, on the other hand, you can objectively say that your feelings of anger are realistic, then the next step is to decide how you are going to deal with them properly.

How do you deal with them appropriately? You have already begun! By working through the first three steps, you have received information that will be very helpful in your efforts to deal with your anger.

THOUGHTS CAN MAKE YOU ANGRY

In the past, it was mistakenly believed that there were only two possible ways to deal with anger: to keep it inside or to let it out.

But what about a third possibility? Remember before when we talked about defusing that stick of dynamite? Our anger is a result of the way we think! In our minds, we are actually interpreting those events that lead to anger. If we can change the way we interpret events and reorganize our thinking patterns, is it possible to stop creating the anger that we feel? Of course! We can learn to control our thoughts *before* they make us angry, regardless of what the events are. Ask yourself this question: Would something that makes you angry make everybody angry? No. The reason why you are angry is because of the way you think about, or interpret, the event. There are some people who would not be angry because they would not interpret the event in a way that would make them so. For example, let's say you've made a doctor's appointment, Ten minutes before you are ready to leave, the receptionist calls to cancel, saying she'll reschedule the appointment at another time. You might be furious, because you feel you should have received more notice, and because you really wanted to be seen. How aggravating! But others might not interpret it that way, and might not get the least bit angry. So if we can learn to interpret events in a more positive, constructive, and calm manner, we can reduce feelings of anger. We wouldn't have to decide whether we wanted to let anger out or keep it inside, because by controlling our thoughts, anger would not even exist most of the time.

You've already completed one of the first steps in reorganizing your thoughts to prevent anger. You've learned that anger can be good and constructive. It can help you to solve problems, and you don't have to be afraid of it. Just becoming aware of its positive elements can help you to be less afraid of anger. This can help you to deal with the thoughts that make you angry.

Good Angry Thoughts Versus Bad Angry Thoughts

Writing down what you think is making you angry can be very helpful. Good angry thoughts can move you to positive, constructive action. You might want to plan your strategies for resolving the problem. On the other hand, many of your thoughts may include so much anger and be so destructive that you feel like banging your head against the wall. Be honest when writing down your thoughts, regardless of how violent or profane they may be. Such rich, colorful language can be helpful in getting your feelings out. This will ultimately help you to control your anger. Try to look at these thoughts more objectively, the way someone else might look at them. Attempt to bring them down to a more manageable level.

Mental Movies

An interesting technique that can be helpful in controlling anger is imagery, or "watching movies in your mind." When you become angry, you frequently have all kinds of pictures in your head of what is making you angry and what you'd like to do to deal with it. These movies can be very helpful.

For example, imagine that you are very, very tired. Your friend calls to tell you that her car has broken down. Could you please pick up her dry cleaning? When you tell her that you are too tired to go, she says something about how she can never depend on you for anything. This is a friend? You are furious. At that moment, imagine all the abusive things that you would like to say to her, and imagine the shocked expression on her face. If you ask her to hold on for a moment, and close your eyes and imagine this as if you were actually doing it, you'll probably be able to complete the phone call without destroying a friendship. You may even smile or laugh as you think about the scenes that are playing through your mind. More about imagery in Chapter 14, "Pain."

Nora was quite fed up with her son, Pesty Pete. Whenever she asked for his help with normal household chores, his answers were fresh and abusive. Just before she was about to give him a haircut with a meat cleaver, she remembered the mental movie technique. She imagined herself strangling him—his eyeballs popping out and gurgling sounds coming from his throat. This helped to get rid of the intense, angry feelings that were making her crazy, and allowed her to deal with Pete more constructively. (No, she's not in jail.)

The Big Red Stop Sign

Another technique that can help you control anger is referred to as "thought stopping." Remember: It is the thoughts in your mind that are making you angry. These are the thoughts you have when you interpret an event. When you find that angry thoughts have come into your head, picture a big red stop sign. Seeing that picture in your mind will serve as a momentary distraction. Then concentrate on something you enjoy, whether it is a peaceful, relaxing scene, a type of food that you like to eat, an activity that you enjoy, or a movie or television program. Whatever you choose, you will divert your thinking and have a better chance of dissipating your anger. You could also participate in a pleasant, distracting activity, such as reading a book, taking a walk, or calling a friend, which will also help you to feel less angry.

Change Your Requirements

People often get angry when they want certain things to occur in certain ways. When your specific requirements are not met, you may feel angry. Trying to modify your requirements can help you to cope with anger.

Let's say that you're not feeling well and you decide to call your doctor. The answering service tells you that he is not in the office and that you should get a return call within a half-hour. When he has still not returned your call after forty-five minutes, you are fuming. Why? Because your requirement of a call back within thirty minutes has not been met. Revise your requirement. Tell yourself that you would have liked a call within thirty minutes, but your doctor may be tied up on another case, in transit, or unable to get to a phone. You'll be satisfied if you get a call at his earliest convenience. By modifying the requirement, you can feel less angry.

Another way to benefit from this technique is to write down those thoughts indicating what your requirements are. Then try to write down new, more flexible desires. This will make you feel better.

PUT YOURSELF IN THEIR SHOES

One of the best ways of dealing with anger toward somebody else is to try to understand exactly what that person is feeling, what the person wants, and why the person is saying what he or she is saying. This will make you more aware of why somebody else is behaving or talking the way he or she is, and you will be better able to deal with it constructively. This will also help you to understand how the other person would feel if he or she was the target of your abusive release of anger.

LET IT OUT LESS EXPLOSIVELY

We have discussed a number of ways to control your thinking and improve your ability to interpret events in ways that do not allow anger to develop. But what if this doesn't always work? What if there are times when you remain as angry as you were before? What can be done to deal with anger constructively when it already exists?

Talk, Don't Bite

Obviously, it is much more desirable to have a constructive discussion over an issue than it is to have an angry exchange of heated words, which accomplishes nothing. In most cases, anger arises from a conflict or problem with another person. Therefore, it is frequently helpful to improve your ability to get your point across constructively. If you are trying to negotiate a better resolution to a problem that may exist between you and somebody else, having a heated argument or "fighting fire with fire" is not the answer. Instead, you want to fight the fire by dousing it and reducing the heatedness of the argument. Try complimenting the person or looking for the positive things in what that person is saying to you, even if you're angry. This works in two ways. One, it will probably surprise the person; and two, you'll be focusing on words or thoughts that are more constructive, rather than letting yourself get angry because of what's being said. Calmly restate your feelings.

Let's take the previous example where you were upset about your friend's demands to pick up the dry cleaning. Instead of blowing up at her and telling her that she is so inconsiderate and just doesn't understand, tell her she's right in calling you. You're glad she thought of you. But then let her know that as much as you would like to do this favor for her, you don't have the strength to even get dressed. Keep looking for something positive to respond to regardless of what she says, and continue to calmly indicate that you don't feel well. Eventually, you'll get the point across, and although she may not be too happy about it (she may even get angry), you will have been able to resolve a problem in a constructive way, with much less anger.

Get Involved in an Activity

In general, one of the best outlets for releasing angry energy is physical activity. Because of lupus, though, this outlet may not be as available to you as you'd like. Besides being angry about something else, the most frustrating aspect of having lupus is that you may be able to participate only in reduced amounts of physical activity. Because you may be prone to fatigue and have less energy, this outlet may not be readily usable. Interestingly, it has been found that physical energy from anger can be released by watching things. For example, by watching a sporting event, you aren't releasing energy through participation in the sport, but you may still be able to "get into it" and reduce your anger that way. Or try watching a particularly violent or emotionally draining movie. You can become so absorbed in the picture that the energy building up from anger is released through worry, fear, or excitement. A movie or book that allows you to identify with the characters, or where the characters allow a release of anger, can be beneficial as well.

A common and very effective outlet for anger, especially among children, is crying. I'm sure you've heard of the therapeutic effects of a good cry. However, this technique is not for everyone. People who can be more open in expressing their emotions may be better able to benefit from this outlet.

Some people like to count to ten when they are angry. This can distract them from what is making them angry, giving them a chance to calm down and think about the situation more constructively. Try counting to a thousand, if necessary!

LET US REVIEW

It is very important to remember that events alone do not make you angry. It is your thoughts—your interpretations of events—that lead to anger. Even if something really terrible happens, it is the meaning that you give to this particular event that makes you angry. It is the way you think about this horrible event that creates your anger. Since your thinking makes you angry, you are responsible for feeling this way. Therefore, you can be just as responsible for changing your way of thinking so that you may cope with your anger, or at least reduce your anger to a more manageable level.

Probably the best way to handle anger is to be in control so that it doesn't build up in the first place. But if it does, remember that if anger is channeled and used constructively, it does have its benefits. Uncontrolled anger can be an unpleasant, negative, destructive emotion. Your efforts are best spent in trying to figure out how to reorganize your thinking so that your anger doesn't get out of hand.

9

Guilt

Have you ever felt guilty? Many individuals with lupus say that they have. Guilt is a very unpleasant emotion. Take the case of Laura, a 34-year-old mother of three. She was very unhappy because she couldn't be the kind of mother she wanted to be. Why not? Well, because she couldn't participate in enough activities with her kids. She wasn't able to give them the amount of time that she wanted to. Frequently, when they asked her to do things with them or to play with them, she couldn't because of her lupus. She wasn't able to accompany them on school field trips, or to take them to the beach. So having lupus made her feel guilty because she felt that she was being a bad mother. Hard to cope? You bet! Let's take a look at what leads to guilty feelings.

THE TWO COMPONENTS OF GUILT

Feelings of guilt usually have two components. The first of these is the "wrongdoing"; you feel that you have done something wrong, or that you haven't done something that you should have done. The second component is the "self-blame"; you blame yourself for doing this wrong thing, and *feel* that you are "bad" because of it. That's the culprit! It is the concept of "badness" that creates the feelings of guilt. It is normal and understandable if you feel bad about doing something wrong. But when you start telling yourself that you *are* bad, guilt follows. What if other people tell you, "It's O.K. You didn't do anything wrong." This may not help. Your feelings of guilt may have nothing to do with what others tell you or what they think. Even if they disagree with you, you may still feel the way you do. Remember: Your guilt comes from the feeling that you are a bad person, rather than from feeling bad about what you have done. Is it fitting to label yourself as a bad person or to blame yourself because you've done something wrong? Even if you have done something wrong, it's better to label that particular behavior rather than yourself as bad.

Is the behavior that you are blaming yourself for really that terrible or wrong? Does it justify the feeling of badness that leads to guilt? In Laura's case, she felt guilty because of her lupus. Does that make sense? Did she make it happen? Of course not. Laura might feel better, therefore, if she emphasized the quality rather than the quantity of time spent with her children.

FALLING SHORT OF EXPECTATIONS

Guilt feelings about their inability to handle their children or the lack of time they have to spend with their children are very common for mothers with lupus. On the other hand, men tend to feel more guilty about their inability to advance in their careers or to fulfill their job responsibilities the way they feel they should. How about Jack, a 48-year-old husband and father of two. He felt guilty because he was not able to work as hard at his job as he used to. He therefore earned less money—not enough to provide for all of the luxuries he and his family would have enjoyed on his old salary. Feeling pressured, Jack tried to work harder to earn more money, which in turn made him feel worse physically. This created feelings of guilt. He felt less capable of being the breadwinner in the family, and consequently believed he was a bad father and husband. How can you cope with these feelings?

Do you see a difference between the way you are doing something and the way you think you should be doing it? If so, you may really feel guilty! How do you work this out? Major union/management problems would be easier to solve! Can you work harder or do more? If you can, then do it. If not, try examining your day-to-day goals for working and living. Check to see if these goals are practical, considering what you can and cannot do because of your lupus. Try to take more pride in what you can do. Although most people hate hearing, "Things could be worse," this phrase is quite true. You might not be able to do anything at all. If you concentrate on the things you can do, and place less emphasis on what you can't, your feelings of guilt will diminish. You'll feel a lot better. Changing the emphasis in your thinking will also help you to lessen the gap between what is and what ought to be. This is what led to the guilty feelings in the first place.

Does this approach work only for working men? No. It applies to anyone who feels guilty about falling short of expectations and de-sires. Barbara, a 16-year-old student, was feeling guilty because she was unable to devote the amount of time to her schoolwork she used to, or because she couldn't spend as much time on it as she would have liked. She was more and more reluctant to go to school because she was so frequently unprepared for her classes, and she missed a number of school days because of lupus. The guilt she felt affected her schoolwork even more. How might Barbara cope with these guilty feelings? It might be beneficial for Barbara to speak to each of her teachers and explain how lupus was affecting her, cautioning her teachers that physical problems might restrict her from devoting the same amount of time to her schoolwork as she had previously, and that her attendance might not be as good as it had been. At that point, it would be helpful to discuss possible methods for making up for this, such as extra projects that she might be able to work on when she was feeling up to it, or alternate arrangements for testing (to try to show her teachers that even with less time available for studying, she was still interested in succeeding in class). By working with her teachers and setting more realistic goals, the feelings of guilt related to having lupus and its effect on her schoolwork should decrease.

TALK IT OVER

It is very important to discuss how you feel about your condition with others who may be affected by it. It is helpful to talk over feel-ings with the important people in your life, to share concerns, and to try to figure out solutions to problems. Janet, a 23-year-old woman who had been married less than a year, had enjoyed a very active so-cial life before developing lupus. In addition to going out on week-ends, she and her husband had played tennis with friends or had participated in other social activities at least two or three evenings during the week. Now, because of the way lupus was affecting her, she had to restrict her activities. She just couldn't go out as fre-quently. She couldn't even play tennis at all. Sometimes, she wouldn't want to go out even once during an entire week. Not only did she feel unhappy about her condition, but she felt extremely guilty about holding her husband back. She felt that he couldn't have a good time because of her. It would be helpful for Janet to discuss alternatives with her husband. If she could arrive at a solution with her husband's cooperation, she could effectively reduce guilt feelings and improve her marriage.

THOUGHTS CAN HURT, TOO

So far, we have been discussing how doing the wrong thing can lead to guilt. But it's not only behavioral mistakes that can lead to guilty feelings. Thoughts can also become upsetting enough to lead to guilt.

Sometimes, you may feel guilty without having done anything wrong. You may merely be thinking things that cause guilt. Pam, a 29-year-old mother of three young children, was feeling terribly guilty. Why? Her 30-year-old husband was spending many hours taking care of the kids and helping her with the housework. Pam knew that her condition meant that she couldn't do what she used to, but she felt bad because her husband had to do so much. She was afraid that he would eventually start complaining. Should Pam blame herself and feel guilty because of her condition?

Dora, a 31-year-old woman with two children, said that she felt guilty because her 64-year-old mother was spending so much time taking care of her and her kids. Dora felt guilty because she was not getting any better and did not know how much longer it would be necessary for her mother to take care of her, and because her father was complaining about the loss of time spent with his wife. Is it appropriate for Dora to blame herself and feel guilty because of a disease she cannot control? Since she hasn't done anything wrong, Dora can feel better if she modifies her thinking.

In order to successfully cope with guilt, you must first focus on what has led to the feelings of guilt. Have you actually done something wrong? Have you really neglected something you shouldn't have? You may feel guilty about your thoughts or desires, rather than specific actions or behaviors. Recognize that if you haven't done anything to justify your feelings of guilt, then you should identify those thoughts that are making you feel like a bad person. Change them. If you can learn to talk to yourself in a positive way, looking at your thoughts objectively and constructively, guilt can be reduced.

Frequently, as in Pam's or Dora's case, feeling guilty is related to seeing yourself as responsible for the actions or behaviors of others.

The more responsible you feel, the more guilt you may feel, especially if you cannot fulfill your responsibility. Frequently, just asking the question, "Why do I feel responsible?" will point out that your thinking is unrealistic. That alone can help to reduce guilt. This is another reason why discussions with others are helpful. They may explain why taking the responsibility for someone else is inappropriate. Be sure to place feelings of responsibility in proper perspective. There is a limit as to how responsible you should feel for someone else's actions or feelings. You are not responsible for having lupus, or for any restrictions this may place on you. Pam should recognize that nobody was forcing her husband to take over the household responsibilities, and Dora should recognize the same thing about her mother. Pam's husband and Dora's mother both decided what they wanted to do. Neither Dora nor Pam should feel responsible for these choices; being aware of this can reduce guilt. Realize that when individuals are not forced to do something, they participate out of choice and desire. The same holds true for your actions. You are reading this book out of choice and desire, aren't you?

"SHOULD" THOUGHTS

Among the most common causes of guilt are thoughts containing the word "should." "Should" is a dirty word! Examples of such thoughts are, "I *should* have been able to finish that job today," "We *should* have that party. All our friends have entertained us this year," "You *should* have let me do the dishes," and "I *shouldn't* have any more pain." These "should" thoughts imply that you must be just about perfect, and on top of everything. When there is a difference between what you feel should occur and what actually does occur, guilt can result. You will become upset whenever you fall short of what you think you should do. Should thoughts lead to guilt simply because they are not sensible, realistic, or justifiable? Should you blame yourself because you have set goals that you may not be able to fulfill?

Now that I've explained what you shouldn't do, what exactly should you do? In order to feel better and reduce feelings of guilt, it is helpful to reword your thoughts to eliminate "should" thoughts. Try to use less demanding words. Say, "It would be nice if I could finish that job today, but I can't," rather than, "I should finish that job today." If your physical condition is restricting your activities, you'll feel much more guilty when "should" thoughts remind you of unfulfilled obligations. If you have trouble changing the wording of your "should" thoughts, try asking yourself, "Why should I . . . ?" or "Who says I should . . . ?" or "Where is it written that I should . . . ?" This may help you decide whether you are setting up impossible requirements for yourself. It can also help you to reduce your feelings of guilt.

Let's say, for example, that you are thinking of having a party because all your friends have invited you to get-togethers. Ask yourself why you should have one? Is it because the "Party Rulebook" tells you so? If you don't have a party, will your friendship license be revoked? If you don't have a party, won't your friends (some friends!) invite you to their homes anymore? As you think about the realistic answers to these questions, it will be easier to realize that you don't have to have a party. Although giving a party would have been a nice gesture, it is more acceptable to wait until you feel better.

THE CONSEQUENCES OF GUILT

So far, we've been discussing what leads to guilt, how you may feel, and how you can try to adjust your thoughts and behaviors to feel better. But what happens if you have not yet been successful in eliminating guilt? People who feel guilty frequently act in negative ways to hide from these feelings. There may be a tendency to indulge in "escape" behaviors, such as drinking or excessive sleeping, which do not deal with problems head-on but, instead, attempt to push them away.

Jill, a 20-year-old secretary, felt guilty because she had stopped making plans with her friends. She had done this because she was embarrassed about how many times she had to cancel plans at the last minute because of her lupus. She felt that since she had had to cancel so often and would probably have to continue to do so, why should she even bother to make plans? As a result, she began to lose friends, and her guilt became more and more difficult for her to bear. She began drinking each day, and going to bed right after dinner, in an attempt to "escape" and to forget her misery. This behavior did not help the situation, and it certainly didn't help her medical condition. In fact, it was downright dangerous. Not only did it compound the problem, but there was the added danger of mixing alcohol and medication. Now Jill had something else to feel guilty about: her escape behavior. This could increase her belief that she was a bad person and lead to even more guilt, creating a vicious cycle.

The first step toward improvement is to look past the escape behavior and identify whatever is causing the guilt. Consider what can be done to rectify the problem causing the guilt. At the same time, try to eliminate any escape behavior, recognizing that it is only a cop-out. It is possible, however, for there to be no clear-cut solution to the events or feelings creating guilt. If, for example, Jill's physical condition is keeping her from making plans with her friends, can she believe that the only way to make things better is to force herself to do things she physically shouldn't? Should she wait to make plans until her lupus "goes away"? That would be ridiculous. Don't give up because no complete solution exists. Look for partial solutions. These may not be as desirable, but they can still help to reduce guilt by reminding you that you are trying to improve the situation. Jill's lupus won't go away, but she could at least try to make small, nondemanding plans with a few friends. And, she certainly could try to explain the problem to her friends so she'd be less embarrassed if she did have to cancel plans.

OTHER SUGGESTIONS

We've talked a lot about how thoughts and behaviors can cause guilt. But what if you feel guilty and can't remember what you were thinking or doing to make you feel that way? How can you start using all these great thought-changing ideas if you don't remember what thoughts you want to change? Good question! In order to identify those "target" thoughts or behaviors, you might want to keep a brief log of feelings or activities that may have caused your guilt. Once you have written these things down, you can then begin figuring out how to change them, improve your outlook, and reduce your guilt.

Mary, aged 39, had been feeling increasingly guilty recently but didn't really know why. By keeping a log, she noticed that besides complaining of fatigue almost all the time, she had been arriving at work late on a regular basis. She wasn't aware of how frequently she had been late, and she had always been proud of her punctuality. The log helped her to see that she needed to improve her morning routine in order to be more punctual. As she worked on this problem, her guilt lessened.

What about those negative thoughts that lead to guilt? It can be very helpful to try to turn these thoughts around, making them more positive and guilt free. For example, let's say that you feel guilty because you believe you are a bad parent. Ask yourself if you have ever done anything that a good parent might do. Just about every parent can come up with something. This starts the process of eliminating your "bad parent blues." The idea is to turn your mind's negative thoughts into reasonable, positive ones. This way, the feeling of guilt will not take a strangle hold!

A FINAL GUILTY THOUGHT

Guilt is a very destructive emotion—one that can certainly interfere with your success in coping with lupus. By become aware of how guilt develops, you have a much better chance of effectively employing coping strategies to reduce guilt and its negative effects.

10

Stress

What is stress? Stress is a response that occurs in your body. It helps you mobilize your strength to deal with different things happening in your life. Many things occur each day that require you to adapt. These are the "stressors." All the changes that occur in your body when something (the stressor) provokes you are known as the "stress response."

With lupus you may experience stress for many reasons. For example, pain alone can cause stress. Your concern about how your disease will affect you can cause stress. Worries about not being able to fulfill responsibilities can be stressful. Problems with medication are also stressors. Any one of these—and more—can provoke the stress response.

IS STRESS GOOD OR BAD?

A certain amount of stress in normal and necessary. Stress helps you to "get your act together," and prepares you to handle your life in the best possible way. Now you're probably thinking, "So why do I always hear people talking about how stress can be harmful?" When people talk about the harmful effects of stress, they are referring to situations in which there is *too much* stress. In those situations, the stress can become destructive. If left unchecked, it can eat away at you and drain all of your energy.

Reasonable amounts of stress can be handled. In fact, they can even be helpful. This chapter, however, is concerned with harmful stress—the kind that can hurt you if it is not controlled. The word "stress" is used very frequently these days. It describes those things that create nervousness, anxiety, tension, anger, or an upset feeling. Even though these are all possible reactions to or causes of stress, they are not synonymous. In other words, they each may result from or cause the stress response.

Esther, a 38-year-old housewife, was under pressure. Her husband was bringing his boss home for dinner. She had just gotten over a flare, and because she knew she got exhausted easily, she carefully paced herself as she prepared the meal so she wouldn't get run-down. The stress she felt was tolerable; that is, until the phone rang. Her husband called to tell her that due to an emergency business meeting that evening, they'd be arriving two hours early! Esther's stress was no longer tolerable!

WHO FEELS STRESS?

Everyone experiences stress. Nobody escapes it. But since stress can be positive or negative, learning how to respond positively will lead to more stable emotional and physical states. If you have a hard time responding to stress, this won't be easy. Some people are more vulnerable to negative stress responses than others. Are you?

THE STRESS RESPONSE

Every person has a unique way of responding to stress. Stress management (effectively managing the way you respond to stress) is within your reach. Your pattern of response depends on a number of things: your upbringing, your self-esteem, your beliefs about yourself and the world, what you say to yourself, and how you guide yourself in your thoughts and actions. The degree to which you feel in control of your life plays a role in your stress response. The way you feel physically and emotionally and the way you get along with people are also a part of it. To sum it up, everyone's method of dealing with stress is unique, depending upon a complex combination of thoughts and behaviors.

Stressor + Interpretation = Stress Response

The way that you respond to stress depends on the "chemistry" between two factors. The first factor is the stressor, or the outside pressures. What is going on around you that is creating the reactions? The second factor is what is within you, or how you interpret things. It is the interaction of the stimulus and your own internal reaction that determines how you respond to stress. (Sound familiar? Yes, it's the same "formula" that can be applied to anger, depression, and all the other emotions.)

This equation has important implications for coping with stress when you realize that it isn't just the environment that causes your response, but also the way you interpret the stressor. Some stressors in the environment would produce stress in anybody. What would happen, for example, if somebody pointed a knife at your throat? Calm acceptance or a stress response? Get the point? It's important to learn how to reduce the number of stressors that negatively affect you, and to improve your reaction to those you can't avoid.

Body Versus Mind

How do you respond to stress? Like your response to anger and other mobilizing emotions, there are two main ways: physically and cognitively. A cognitive response includes the way you think and feel. Most people respond to stress in both ways, although it is possible for you to respond in only one way.

What happens physically? If you experience a stressful situation, the circulatory system speeds up. Blood is pushed rapidly toward different parts of the body, particularly those parts necessary to protect you. Because the blood supply is diverted toward these essential parts, the supply to the digestive system is usually reduced. As a result, the digestive process slows down, making it work less efficiently.

Your may tremble or perspire. Your face may flush. You may feel a surge of adrenaline flowing through your body. Your mouth may become dry or you may feel nauseated. Your breathing may become more rapid and shallow. Your heart may begin to pound. Your muscles may become tight, creating headaches, cramps, or other painful reactions. Sounds lovely, doesn't it?

You may be vulnerable to stress in your own unique way. Certain parts of your body may tend to be more vulnerable to the effects of stressors. For example, have you ever felt extreme intestinal discomfort from stress, and automatically clutched your stomach? Or have you ever endured a painful headache? There is a possibility that stress may have even played a role in lupus, or in another illness or condition that you've suffered.

Chronic or prolonged stress puts a severe strain on your body. When your body is strong, it can fight off most foreign invaders, bac-

teria, and germs. As a result, many diseases can be avoided. But prolonged stress puts such a strain on the body that your defense
mechanisms may break down. This, in turn, makes your body more
vulnerable to the very problems you'd like to avoid!

Have you heard of the "fight or flight" syndrome? Animals do this
when they feel threatened. The animal either prepares to fight or runs
away, a purely physical response. You will not see an animal hesitate,
scratch his head, and think about what should be done! But humans
have the unique ability to think and reason! Lucky us! So we include
cognitive responses in our repertoire. (By the way, researchers feel
that this is one of the main reasons why human beings are susceptible
to so much stress-related physical illness. By thinking instead of acting, we may not be dealing with stress as effectively as we might.)

When does stress lead to physical problems? When you can't respond to stress in a way that eliminates it, the stress continues unabated. Being unable to do anything about it may cause even more
stress, creating a vicious cycle. This can take its toll on your body.

Your cognitive or emotional response to stress may not be as visible.
You may not be able to concentrate as well, as your attention span is reduced. Consequently, you may have trouble learning something new.
You may be afraid to do things. You may withdraw or feel nervous. You
may lose confidence in yourself. As you become aware of unpleasant
physical responses to stress, you may feel even more stressed. For example, if you feel stress and respond with shallow, rapid breathing or
heart palpitations, your awareness of these physical responses may create even more stress. This can lead to feelings of panic.

THREE RESPONSES TO STRESS

When a stressful stimulus occurs, you will most likely respond in one
of three ways. You might respond immediately and impulsively without giving enough thought to a better response. You might not respond at all, and either try to ride it out or become so frozen that you
are unable to respond. Finally, you may respond to stressors in a well-
planned, organized, and effective manner. If so, you may not even
need this chapter! But if not, read on!

HOW TO DEAL WITH STRESS

Remember: Stress can be managed and controlled, but it cannot be
eliminated. Stress will always exist. You can learn to deal with differ-

ent amounts and kinds of stress, but you'll never be able to make stress go away. For a person with lupus, it is especially important that stress be controlled. Why? Although stress by itself does not cause lupus, it certainly may play a role in exacerbating your lupus symptoms.

Let's begin by mentioning the wrong ways of responding to stress. These are the ways that won't help you: smoking, getting drunk, using drugs, overeating, and overactivity. Not only will these activities distract you and delay the effects of stress, but they can also hurt you.

So what should you do? Try to learn new, more appropriate ways of dealing with stress than the methods you've been using.

Relaxation Procedures

The best way to start controlling stress is by using relaxation procedures. Try the "quick release" method discussed in the introductory chapter of this section. Other successful methods of relaxation include meditation, self-hypnosis, imagery, and even a warm shower! Deep breathing alone can help to eliminate tension from the body, slow down the heart, and create a greater sense of well-being. Learning to relax can be helpful in reducing the amount of stress you are experiencing. It will give your body a chance to rest and recuperate as well. A stronger body can deal more effectively with the ravages of stress (or of life)! Have you been experiencing any difficulties sleeping since the onset of your condition? Relaxation will help you to sleep better.

Pinpointing Stressors

Stress is a type of energy that needs release. It can be handled positively or negatively. Stress is negative when you cannot handle it well. In order to learn how to cope successfully, you must first identify your stressors. What, specifically, is causing you to feel stress? Are you concerned about medication? Do you fear another flare? Are you having a hard time dealing with pain or the other symptoms of lupus? Perhaps you're concerned about the reactions of others. These are all possible lupus-related stressors, and, of course, there are plenty more.

What if you're not sure what's causing your stress? How can you figure out what it is? One way is to keep a record of your activities and experiences, using numerical ratings such as those in a scale called the SUD scale. SUD stands for subjective units of disturbance. How does it work? Ratings on this scale range from 0 to 100, depending on the amount of stress you're experiencing. Use 100 to represent the most extreme and disturbing stress, and 0 to represent no stress (total and complete relaxation). Then rate your activities and experiences on the SUD scale. The ones with the higher SUD numbers are the ones causing you the most stress. For example, loud, blasting music from your teenager's radio might be rated a whopping 85!

Identifying Your Stress Reactions

Once you have begun identifying your stressors, you must then become completely aware of your responses to them. Are they more physiological or psychological? What parts of your body seem to be the most vulnerable? What kind of reaction does your body show? Does your attention span suffer? Do you start losing confidence, or feel as if you're slipping? As you become more aware of the changes that occur, you will develop a more complete picture of your unique stress response. You'll be able to recognize the stressors that affect you and how you react to them. You'll then be better able to decide whether you should modify your behavior in response to the stressor.

What's the next step? Once you have recognized which stressors are negative, try to determine whether you can eliminate them. If you can, start figuring out how to do it. Removing the source of stress is an obvious and logical way to manage stress. Develop a plan of attack. This might include a number of alternative strategies, all designed to remove or minimize the impact of the stressor. Taking a sledgehammer to that radio might be great, if you could lift the hammer!

But what happens if you can't eliminate the source of your stress? You'll then have to work on your means of interpreting what's going on. You'll have to work on your thinking and your responding in order to manage stress. In such cases, changing the stressor is out of your control, but changing the way you react isn't. You might want to use some of the suggestions discussed in Chapters 6 and 8. The use of systematic desensitization, which was discussed in Chapter 7, "Fears and Anxieties," can also be beneficial. Many techniques for changing your thinking have already been discussed in previous chapters.

Relieving Physical Stress

Certain physical activities can be great for stress control. For example, some people can relieve tension or stress by driving. As long as the driver continues to observe safety rules, driving can be very relaxing.

Exercising

Another important way of dealing with stress is by exercising. As you'll read later, exercise not only is important in helping you deal with stress, but can also be a very healthy component of your treatment program for lupus. Regardless of how lupus is affecting you, there are still exercises you can do to help yourself control stress. Virtually any type of exercise can be effective. Anything that gets the body moving, gets the heart pumping faster, and allows for a release of tension is ideal.

Keeping Busy the Fun Way

Hobbies and other leisure activities can be very helpful. They can divert your attention away from the stressful situation, directing it toward something more enjoyable. These activities will also help you feel productive. A lack of productivity may be one of the stressors giving you problems in the first place!

Another technique for dealing with stress is sleep. Some people have difficulty sleeping when experiencing high levels of stress; this applies to those with lupus and those on medication. However, you may not be one of those people and might be able to take naps to reduce stress.

IN CONCLUSION

What are your goals? If stress is interfering with your achievement of these goals, then your stress response is negative. Learning how to control stress is a very necessary part of successfully achieving your goals, as well as successfully coping with lupus.

11

Other Emotions

The emotions we've covered so far in this section are not the only ones, of course. Worry, for example, is a basic emotion. What might you worry about? Have you got a month to discuss all the possibilities? You've probably worried about the future, what your life will be like, whether your medication will ever be reduced, and how your life will change because of lupus, among countless other things. What other emotions enter into the picture? This chapter will discuss five other emotions common for people with lupus: boredom, envy, loneliness, upset, and grief.

BOREDOM

Hopefully, by this time, you are not so bored that you have stopped reading! As long as you aren't bored, let's talk a little about boredom! What an empty feeling! It's one of the worst feelings anyone can experience. It has been said that more problems and serious tragedies come from being bored than from any other single condition.

Why are you bored? There may be no meaningful activity going on, no stimulation or excitement. Your life may seem to be going nowhere. Nothing is challenging you, and there's no incentive to do anything. Because you weren't born bored, you must have learned to be bored. You weren't always bored, and even now you are not always bored. There are still certain things that hold your attention from time to time. Right?

Is Lupus Boring?

I bet you never thought of lupus as boring. But it can be, primarily because of any restrictions your condition may impose on you. Many activities that provided enjoyment for you in the past may now be out of reach. You may not even want to bother starting something new, telling yourself that future activities will be restricted because of lupus.

Celia was too tired to leave her house. She couldn't go shopping, she couldn't meet friends for lunch, and she was fed up with the garbage on television. Was Celia bored? You bet she was! Her friend suggested that Celia go along with her to take a course in interior decorating, since Celia had a lot of talent in this field. But despite her enthusiasm, she decided not to because she didn't want to start something she felt she couldn't finish.

Olive hated the fact that her condition prevented her from knitting. She was tired of music, and she didn't want to read. Was Olive bored? Definitely! But did she have to be bored? No! Her family and friends suggested that she try new activities, and Olive was soon able to feel less bored.

So what should you do? Don't let your condition cause you to give up living. Distinguish between what you can do and what you can't. You may have to curtail some activities or drop one or two of them because of lupus. But you don't have to eliminate all activities from your life simply because you feel you won't complete them.

"Unboring" Yourself

What can you do about your boredom? The first step is to analyze why you are bored. What is causing the boredom? Obviously, figuring this out will help you to determine how you can improve things. Then you'll want to see what you can do to add some interest to your life. But don't feel that you must push yourself to enjoy something. Forcing yourself to become amused rarely works. You may find that activities you used to enjoy have become artificial and uninteresting. You may no longer get any pleasure from them. That doesn't mean, however, that you should give up and not try to do something. Trying some new activities will make your life more interesting. Don't limit yourself to those things that used to interest you. Preferences change. Try things that never interested you before, because they might now spark an interest in you.

Learn Something New!

One of the most effective weapons against boredom is learning. The mind is like a sponge, and is always ready and willing to soak up more information and knowledge. Select a potentially interesting topic you don't know much about. Try to learn something about it. You may want to begin by simply going to the library and reading some books on the topic. Perhaps you'd like to enroll in an adult education course. Boredom often disappears quickly once you are involved in something new. Learning is a great way to relieve boredom.

You can also become bored if your social life is suffering. What can you do about this? Once again, try to learn something, especially by taking courses of some kind. Aside from the mental stimulation you'll get from such learning activities, you may also meet interesting and challenging people. Increasing your circle of friends is a good way to fight boredom.

Anticipation!

One of the best ways to fight boredom is to always give yourself something to look forward to. It doesn't matter how small this may be. It can be as simple as reading a chapter of a good book, writing a letter, making that phone call you've been looking forward to, watching a television program you've been excited about, or meeting somebody special for lunch. Try to schedule something to look forward to every day. This way, even if part of your day seems boring, whether you're doing menial chores or just resting to build up your strength, you will at least have something enjoyable to look forward to. You won't give the weeds of boredom a chance to take root!

Goal Setting

Set goals for yourself, both short-term and long-term. Boredom can arise from plodding with no purpose in life. Having something specific and tangible to shoot for can be helpful in fighting boredom. This doesn't mean you'll never be bored. You may still have to give yourself an occasional kick in the derriere to keep moving toward those goals. But isn't it better to have something to shoot for than to have nothing at all?

ENVY

You've heard the cliché, "The grass is always greener . . ." If you have lupus, you are probably envious of others who do not. This is understandable. You may also be envious of other people who are able to do more than you can.

Envy can be a destructive emotion, because it's a type of self-torture. It can be very painful. People who are envious constantly put themselves down and compare themselves with the better qualities of other people. They feel inferior. This can lead to other feelings as well, such as anger or depression.

Why is envy a problem? Because it shows that you are not satisfied with being yourself. You want to be like somebody else. You want to have what somebody else has. Does this mean that the other person has a happy life? Is that person happier than you in every way? You may have lupus, but this doesn't mean that everything else about the other person's life is superior. Stop and think for a moment. I'm sure you can come up with some areas in which your life is better!

Is Envy a Positive Emotion?

In general, emotions usually serve a purpose. Emotions such as anger and anxiety mobilize you to prepare to handle their sources. On the other hand, envy is a destructive emotion. It does not have the positive qualities that other emotions may have. But maybe you can find something positive in envy. If you recognize that you're envious, analyze the reason why. Try to change the way you feel by concentrating on yourself and your own attributes. Don't let envy get you down.

How Does Envy Occur?

Basically, there are four conditions necessary for you to feel envious. First, you feel deprived. You feel like you can't have something that you want or need. This doesn't mean you want only money, pleasure, working joints, and good health. Envy is an intense feeling that involves more than this. It involves a deep feeling of dissatisfaction, unhappiness, and discontent. Second, somebody else has whatever it is that you feel you're missing. Third, you feel powerless to do anything about it. You feel totally unable to change the circumstances that have made you envious in the first place. This helplessness causes you to feel more and more bitter, and this makes you even more envious! Fourth, there is a change in the relationship between you and whatever it is that you envy, be it person, object, or situation. You no longer simply compare yourself with someone else, but feel fiercely competitive with that person. You may begin to feel that the only reason you don't have what you would like is because somebody else does.

If you feel envious, is it necessarily the same kind of envy that everyone feels? No. There are actually two types of envy. One is an envy of tangible things (cars, boats, homes, friends, and so on). The other is an envy of less tangible, abstract things, such as pleasure or health. If you have lupus, you may still have many tangible things. You may still have a family, a car, and a place to live. You may still have a job. But the fact that you're not happy with your medical condition makes you envious.

What Can You Do?

Concentrate on being yourself. Increase the positive benefits and pleasures you can get out of life. Why worry about comparing yourself with somebody else? What's that going to do? Sure, your body may not be functioning the way it used to. But that doesn't mean you can't enjoy life as much as anybody else can. Set up reasonable goals for yourself, considering other things you have and how you feel. Then you can say that you're living your life as enjoyably as anybody else. You will be able to do this when you stop comparing yourself with others. Remember, you are you. Concentrate on making the best of your own life.

LONELINESS

There is a difference between being alone and being lonely. Being alone simply means that there is no one else with you. This can be either good or bad. But being lonely is usually a downer. If you feel lonely, it doesn't really matter whether there's anyone with you. What's more important is your relationship with the people you're with. Loneliness is a sad, empty feeling, but one that is usually created by you.

Why might you feel lonely? You may feel left out if you can't spend time with others the way you used to, either because you're not feeling well or because you can't do what others want to do. Maybe you feel lonely because other people don't want to be with you. You may decide to change some of your relationships because you don't want to risk being rejected. Does this mean that you'll be happy about these changes? No.

It's hard to be lonely. Not just because you feel bad, though. It actually takes effort to make yourself lonely—it doesn't just happen. And you have to work hard to keep yourself feeling lonely. There are many opportunities to be with people. As a result, loneliness usually occurs out of choice rather than by accident. In order to be really lonely, you'd have to purposely exclude everyone around you from your life. You'd always have to be on your guard, protecting yourself from the horrible possibility of making a new friend!

Why Be Lonely?

Why might you want to be lonely? There are four reasons. First, if you're lonely, you probably enjoy being lonely. This may contradict your complaints to everyone else. You're lonely because you like it enough not to do anything about it. Second, if you're lonely, it's because you're hard to please. You may feel that you don't want to bother even trying to create new relationships because no one meets all of your requirements. Third, you may be lonely because you feel you must be lonely. You've resigned yourself to it. You tell yourself that this is part of the price you have to pay for having lupus! Fourth, and probably most important, you may be lonely because you're afraid. You're afraid to develop new relationships. You're afraid to make yourself vulnerable because you fear rejection. You may recall previous experiences that did not work out the way you wanted. You don't want to relive the hurt and pain.

Break Your Lonely Ways

Reading about this isn't easy, especially if you are a lonely person. Why? It's not easy to think that you may have done this to yourself! But there is still a light at the end of the tunnel! Recognize where your feelings of loneliness come from. Admit to yourself that loneliness may not be such a great feeling and that you should try to change it. There are things that you can do.

Don't Be a Pusher

The first step is to stop pushing people away. Your body is sending out signals that tell people that you don't want them around. Your negative body language can reduce your number of acquaintances, adding to your feeling of loneliness. You must stop relaying these messages. You have to learn to give off positive vibrations—the kind that welcome people instead of chasing them away.

Contact!

Once you start giving off new, more positive vibes, you'll want to make more friends. How can you meet people? You can start by getting involved in some kind of organization. This type of activity usually attracts people who are interested in being with others who share a common goal. Because you have lupus, you may want to become involved in your local chapter of the Lupus Foundation. There you'll meet other people with similar concerns who can help you to better cope with your illness. In addition, you may be able to find ways of helping others who have lupus. This is a great way to develop friendships.

Try getting involved in a new learning activity or hobby. Take adult education courses, for example. This will help alleviate loneliness as well as boredom. Invite people to your home, but pace yourself so that you don't become exhausted. Most importantly, be receptive to the people that you meet. Try to see the good in everyone. Don't reject someone simply because there are some things that you don't like.

If you work at conquering loneliness, you'll feel much better about yourself and about your life. Your life will become more enjoyable, despite your having lupus. Give yourself and others a chance, and your feelings of loneliness will disappear, regardless of the limitations your condition has placed on you.

UPSET

Are there times when you are unhappy but not really depressed? Or when you feel uncomfortable but not anxious? You may not know exactly what's bothering you, or what to do about it. Or you may know exactly what's wrong, but you just don't like it. You can do things, but you wish you could feel better. You may feel mixed up, confused, disturbed, agitated, or shaken up. This is typical of feeling upset. Can you get upset because of lupus? Be serious, now!

When things happen to upset you, you may try to push them out of your mind so that you can adjust as slowly and as comfortably as possible. But eventually, you'll certainly want to come to grips with them.

Like other emotions, being upset can propel you to do something. So what should you do when you're all motivated? Try to figure out why you're upset, so you can do something about it. There's probably something in your life that is out of sorts. Things are not moving along smoothly. Something has "upset the apple cart."

Rose was upset. A 34-year-old mother of four, she had just completed her latest car-pool adventure and was about to relax in front of her favorite soap opera on the tube. She had a gnawing feeling that things just weren't right, and this upset her. She knew she was upset when she found that she couldn't enjoy her program. My goodness, she had been hooked on this show for almost twenty years! But she decided to turn off the TV and figure out what was upsetting her. After at least four commercials' worth of thought, she realized that it was her soap opera that was bothering her! She felt that the characters on the program, despite all of their script problems, were better off than she was. They didn't have lupus, but she did! None of them needed medication—only she did! As she thought about it, however, she realized that perhaps she was making something out of nothing. Actors and actresses have their own problems. So what if she also had something she must learn to live with? She had proven to herself that she could live and be happy, even with lupus. She quickly noticed that she was feeling much better. In fact, she was able to turn on the television and breathlessly catch the last few minutes of her show!

Once you discover why you are upset, you can act to resolve your feelings. If you can identify what is upsetting you, then you can plan a strategy to eliminate your distress. However, if you can't figure out what is upsetting you, recognize that you can't and move on.

GRIEF

Grief is usually an unpleasant emotion. Feelings of grief, or mourning over a loss, are common with people who have lupus, especially when they are initially diagnosed. You may grieve the major changes in life necessitated by your lupus. Why do you grieve? Because you're aware that you have lost something that you value: in this case, your former lifestyle. The loss may be temporary or permanent. You may feel that you have lost some physical strength. You may not like yourself as much, and may grieve this feeling of lower self-esteem.

Grief may occur as you sense that your role in life has changed to one of lesser importance. If you are used to having one role within your family, and this role has been modified or significantly changed because of your having lupus, you may grieve this loss. Paul was a 38-year-old construction worker. He took pride in providing a good income for his wife and five children. But then, along came lupus. He was no longer able to work the overtime he had grown accustomed to. There was some concern about his continuing in the construction field at all, and where else he would be able to earn that kind of money. He recognized that his wife was going to have to work to supplement his reduced income. His role as breadwinner was being changed and he was miserable. This change in lifestyle happens frequently for the breadwinner with lupus because of a physical need to change jobs or to adjust to reduced earning capacities because of the condition. The person's role as breadwinner is reduced, if not eliminated, and this can cause grief.

This does not mean that grief is bad. If the feeling of grief develops, it shows that you have something very important that has to be worked through. The feelings that have to be worked through are necessary to adjust to having lupus. What do you do about your grief? It cannot be avoided. Only by thinking about your grief experience will you be able to get past it and get on with your life.

Crying is helpful. That doesn't mean you should force yourself to sob, but if the tears start welling up, don't stop yourself. Let them out. Think about what you've lost, what has changed, and what will change. Talk about your feelings with the people you're close with. Don't avoid facing up to the fact that you have lupus or you won't be able to go through the grieving process. If you want to feel better, you must work through grief. Mourning periods or times of grief don't last forever. Hopefully, you'll be reassured to know that even if you feel absolutely numb or devastated by grief, you're helping yourself by living through it. You will feel better in the future.

Grief is like a deep infection. The only way you can help certain infections get better is by opening them up and letting what's inside ooze out. It may be painful, but eventually the wound will be completely drained so it can begin to heal. See the analogy? Once you have worked through your grief, the healing can begin.

PART III
Changes in General Lifestyle

12

Coping With Changes in General Lifestyle— An Introduction

So you have to make changes in some aspects of your lifestyle because of lupus? Yes, that is all part of the "package." But changes may occur in anyone's life for a number of reasons. If you started a new job, you might have to wake up at a different time, go to work in a new direction by a new form of transportation, or "survive" on a different salary. If your new job required you to move, you would have to meet a whole new group of people. If you got a new car, you'd have to get used to its new gadgets, as well as its quirks. If there was a new addition to the family, you'd have to get used to crying, changing diapers, and night feedings.

In your case, lupus is a new addition to your life! Although it may be hard for you to try to lead a normal life when you know your condition may never be totally cured, you're not (or shouldn't be) aiming for perfection. You just want to feel better, enjoy life, and do what you can. That's reasonable and achievable.

Because lupus can affect work, family life, sexuality, social activities with friends, finances, and other aspects of day-to-day living, it's important for you to learn how to cope with changes in lifestyle. In some cases, these changes may be minimal. But you might as well understand what you can do to cope with any changes that do occur.

Your lifestyle is of your own choosing. You'll automatically take many different factors into consideration when determining what your lifestyle is and what you want it to be. You can decide how full you want your days to be. You may also decide to put things off until you "feel better." But in the case of lupus, why wait? Why not try to see what you can do right now to improve the quality of your life, even while you're learning to live with lupus?

MAKING SOME CHANGES

A good way to change your lifestyle is to look for ways to make things easier for yourself. This may allow you to continue doing much of what you want to do, without putting as much pressure on your body. In fact, as you make changes (at your own pace), you'll feel even better because you'll probably experience less discomfort. Certain lifestyle changes can help you to avoid or reduce discomfort, as well as save your energy.

For example, try to spread your most taxing activities over a reasonable period of time. Why is it necessary to do all the house cleaning in one day? Spread it out. Pace yourself. Make sure you include rest periods during the course of the day so you can "recharge your batteries."

GETTING USED TO THE CHANGES

What are some of the factors that will determine how well you'll adapt to changes in your lifestyle? There are many. For example, what were you doing before you were diagnosed with lupus? How satisfied were you with your major vocational (job) and avocational (leisure or recreation) activities? How much education did you have? How supportive were the people close to you—both family and friends? How has your condition affected you, both physically and emotionally? These and other questions play a role in determining how you'll adjust to lupus, its treatment, and any changes it necessitates. But that doesn't mean your hands are tied. You can improve the way you deal with virtually every aspect of lupus.

Yes, there will be some changes in your lifestyle. But why assume that all of them have to be negative? Isn't it possible that some of them might be for the better? Maybe you were such a hard worker that you never spent enough time with your family. If you have to cut back on your work schedule because of lupus, perhaps you'll enjoy the increased time you'll get to spend with your family. It's possible that some of the medication you'll use to control lupus will also help control other pesty problems that have been troubling you for a while (whether related to lupus or not). Learning to take better care of yourself will pay off in the long run. So don't convince yourself that your life is ruined because you have lupus. Always look at the positive in any situation. We'll be discussing how to deal with as many of the negatives as possible.

Your head may be spinning, fearing changes that may have to take place in your activity schedule, job, or social relationships. You may also be apprehensive about dealing with physical discomfort, body changes, and medication, to name only a few areas of concern. In fact, you may even be concerned that you won't be able to perform your normal chores and responsibilities. This concern is not unusual. Most people with lupus do feel this way. But feelings will improve. Being aware that you can do more will also help improve your spirits.

How About Denial?

What happens if you decide not to comply with necessary changes in lifestyle? This may indicate that you're trying to deny your problem. Denial is a very common coping strategy. But believe it or not, denial can be a positive technique. How? It can be helpful by keeping you from dwelling on problems that aren't helped by dwelling! But denial has its negative side, too. What if denial keeps you from doing what you need to do? For example, what if you don't get enough rest, or you don't pace yourself, or you don't take all your medication, or worse! This is destructive denial, and it can hurt you. Hopefully, the fact that you're reading this book in the first place shows that you're not really denying inappropriately. But continue to stay on top of this.

GUIDELINES FOR CHANGE

Here are some general guidelines for living with lupus that make sense if you need to modify your lifestyle:

- Be aware of how your body feels. How is it reacting to the things you are doing? Act accordingly.
- Build on the talents and activities you can still enjoy (and there'll be plenty of them).
- Pamper yourself a little. Learn that you don't have to do everything for yourself. Accept help from others when necessary and don't push yourself to do anything.
- Be more protective of yourself. Follow normal routines you have established to get the proper amount of sleep, exercise, and nutrition. Avoid contagious diseases, injuries, and infections.

- Remember: You are the most important ingredient in the recipe for successful adjustment to having lupus. Help yourself.

Coping with changes in lifestyle is a very important part of the process we call rehabilitation. What is your goal? To help yourself live as satisfying a life as possible despite your condition.

The rest of this book will address many of your concerns about lifestyle changes. The remaining chapters of Part III will be concerned primarily with changes in the things you do, the way your body feels, and the way lupus affects you. So read on, and let's get your act together!

13

Physical Changes

Caution: Reading this chapter may be hazardous to your health. Your emotional health, that is! Hazardous? Yes, if you start feeling that you're going to experience all the symptoms discussed in the chapter. Please, please, please remember: No one every gets all the symptoms of lupus and most people get only a few. Read this chapter and learn about any symptoms you do have. Don't be frightened when you read about the ones you don't have because you may never get them.

Any chronic illness can affect you in two ways—physically and psychologically. We've discussed how to cope with your emotions; now let's focus on the physical effects of lupus. They can be more noticeable, and they do play a major role in your psychological adjustment to having lupus. In addition, there are lots of possible physical symptoms. You can't do something about all of them, but many of them can be treated with medication, and some of them can also be helped by changing things about yourself or your life. Even then, some symptoms may just persist. With those, you simply must learn to accept them. You must learn to live with them, even if you don't like them. That may seem like a tall order, but what choice do you have? After all, you're still the same person inside. So why not concentrate on the things you *can* do something about? Deal with physical symptoms as they come—one at a time. Don't anticipate the worst, since the worst rarely happens.

Let's discuss some of the more common and troublesome symptoms of lupus. If there's anything you can do about them, suggestions will be offered. If not, at least you'll learn more about the symptoms, and you'll become aware that you're not alone in experiencing them.

JOINT PROBLEMS

One of the first and most common complaints that brings people to physicians, and which may ultimately result in a diagnosis of lupus, is persistently aching joints (especially the wrists, fingers, or knees). These achy joints may lead you to suspect you have arthritis, but arthritis may be only one symptom of lupus.

Joint involvement is considered to be one of the most prevalent symptoms of all. Anywhere from 80–90 percent of all people with lupus will experience joint pain or arthritislike symptoms sometime during the course of their illness. More than half will probably experience muscle aches as well. Joint aches and pains are so common that this is one of the criteria used by physicians in diagnosing lupus.

Which joints can be affected? The pain can occur in the hands, arms, legs, or feet, as well as in the joints—the shoulders, hips, lower jaw, and knees. Often there is a lot of pain even if the joints are not red or swollen.

What Happens?

The joint pain you experience is due to inflammation. This inflammation occurs in the lining of the joints and may cause swelling. Because you never know where the inflammation is going to occur, you can rarely predict which joints are going to end up aching. You may be a good guesser, though, based on your previous experiences!

Joint pain is usually not constant—it comes and goes. However, individual attacks of joint pain may last from several hours to several days or weeks. During this period of time, you can become so sensitive to the way you feel that you may easily begin to predict when the joint pain will be more or less intense.

When does it hurt most? You may notice more intense joint pain or stiffness in the morning when you awaken, or in the evening prior to going to bed. For some reason the symptom tends to be less noticeable during the day, and you may notice improvement in your ability to move the joints comfortably.

Along with the discomfort that is felt, your joints may feel exceptionally tender. It may be painful to even touch the affected joints. Fluid may accumulate, and does so most often in the knees. Redness and warmth of the joints affected with arthritislike symptoms also occur, but not as often as the tenderness. Fortunately, joint involvement in lupus rarely results in a deformity of the joint.

Effects of Joint Involvement on Your Lifestyle

Joint aches and pains are uncomfortable. They can make it harder for you to cope, and changes in lifestyle may be necessary. Walking may be more difficult, and certain physical activities may have to be curtailed when joint symptoms are intense. A positive note: Joint symptoms decrease in intensity as your body responds to treatment for lupus.

Treating Joint Pain

The use of drugs has been helpful in reducing the effects of joint aches and pains. Anti-inflammatory drugs, such as aspirin and other aspirin derivatives, are usually used at first, since arthritis alone is usually not sufficient to justify the use of corticosteroids. If you need steroids for treatment of other symptoms of lupus, the use of these drugs will also improve problems with joints. Surgery is usually not necessary.

A warm (not hot) bath or shower may be helpful. Gentle exercises may help to loosen you up. If you experience any stiffness during the day, work it out of your joints as comfortably as you can.

In a small number of more extreme cases, where joints have lost a good deal of strength or mobility, some people with lupus may use supportive devices, such as canes, splints, braces, crutches, or even walkers. In some cases, they may be helpful for joints such as the hands, ankles, feet, hips, or knees. They preserve and protect them (sounds like the U.S. Constitution!) and allow for as much functional mobility as possible. These devices may also help by spreading out the weight that would be placed on any weight-bearing joints; however, don't feel as if you have to depend on these devices. Discuss their use with your physician to see if there's any benefit to you.

Ischemic Necrosis

A discussion of joint problems would not be complete without referring to ischemic necrosis (which used to be called aseptic or avascular necrosis). It is a condition involving a decrease or loss of blood supply to a particular bone, and it is often uncertain whether ischemic necrosis results from the use of corticosteroids or from lupus activity itself. Either of these two causes may be to blame. It is one of the potentially serious consequences of the combination of inflammation, reduced blood supply, and joint involvement. In extreme cases, it may require surgical replacement of the joint that is affected. Although ischemic necrosis occurs relatively infrequently, it can be serious because it usually involves the weight-bearing joints such as the hips or shoulders, as well as the knees or ankles, since these are the joints that tend to be more affected by loss of blood supply. This is usually the only way in which major bone damage can occur if you have lupus.

RASHES

Rashes clash! They clash with your happiness, they clash with the way you see yourself, and they clash with the way you feel. But unfortunately, rashes are one of the more common symptoms of lupus. They are the major symptom of discoid lupus, but they also are very common in systemic lupus. The classic butterfly rash (redness across the bridge of the nose that spreads out to each cheek below the eyes) has long been one of the most noticeable signs of lupus.

Although the butterfly rash is the most common, rashes may appear anywhere. Arm and leg rashes are almost as common as facial rashes. The rash is usually reddish in color and may or may not be raised and scaly. More than two thirds of all individuals with lupus will eventually have some type of skin rash.

There's no way of knowing how long your rash will last, or how dark the reddish color will be. Rashes or redness are usually more noticeable during flares, and may be less so or may go away altogether during remission. But the rash is not a barometer measuring the intensity of your flare. ("The worse the flare, the more rash there is" is not true!)

Rashes may itch! That can be even more unpleasant than the unsightliness that you dread. Not all rashes are itchy, though. Your itchiness may be caused by something other than a rash. Sometimes dry skin is the culprit. Your skin may be dry because of age, because of lupus, or because of medication that you are taking. The cause of the itchiness determines how it should be treated. If you think medication may be causing the itchiness, check with your physician to see if changes in the dosage can help. Otherwise, applying lubricants or ointments to the skin may be helpful.

Rashes can be upsetting because you may feel that they distort your appearance. You may feel they attract attention to you, but certainly not the kind you want. You may be apprehensive that people will shun you, fearing that your lupus and its rash are contagious. You can tell them about lupus, but they may still be uncomfortable. Therefore, treatment for rashes is important to help you feel better physically as well as emotionally.

Crashing on Rashes

So how are rashes treated? Sandpaper is not the answer! Treatment for rashes involves the use of different types of medications. Corticosteroid creams or ointments are applied and do help. In addition, whatever medication you are taking for the overall control of lupus will help the rash as well. Different types of cosmetic, medical make-up may be used to cover up the rash. This can reduce some of the embarrassment you might feel. A few of them also contain sunblock ingredients—two benefits for the price of one!

FATIGUE

Do you become more tired than you used to more easily? Does your bed seem to be your favorite place in the whole world? If so, you're not alone. Fatigue (yawn!) is one of the most common and debilitating problems for individuals with lupus. Your body simply may not be able to do what you want it to do. Fatigue encompasses the loss of that "get up and go" feeling, not only tiredness or sleepiness. It makes you feel so tired that you just can't complete the things that you want to complete. One of the most upsetting things about fatigue is that you never know when it's going to hit you. You may be going along just fine, and then bang—all of a sudden it feels as if somebody has just pulled the plug! You may awaken in the morning feeling fine; however, fatigue may come on quickly during the day. On the other hand, you may awaken in the morning feeling very tired and find that your energy builds up during the day.

How do you feel when fatigue hits? You feel like a rag doll, with arms and legs that are so floppy and limp that you just can't move them. You feel like a marionette supported by strings, after the strings are cut. You feel like a balloon that has popped and just collapses in a whoosh. Or you quiver and tremble uncontrollably, like a bowl of jello. Whatever it feels like to you, fatigue is hard to deal with.

Unfortunately, the fatigue itself is not your only problem. The disbelief of the people around you will add to your frustration. They may not be able to understand how you can go from being active and on the ball to being tired and listless in such a short period of time.

Louise was playing bridge with her friends. They were sitting and talking over the latest episode of their favorite television program when, seemingly all of a sudden, Louise asked to be excused so she could go and plop on the couch. She couldn't get up, and she weakly asked her friends to help straighten up before they left. Lazy, no. Sleepy, no. Lupus fatigue, yes!

There are two possible reasons for feeling so tired. In some cases you'll feel tired following some activity or expenditure of energy. But the other more puzzling fatigue comes by surprise. Even though you may not have done anything tiring, your body all of a sudden decides to go on a rest cure! You feel as if the energy has drained right out of your body, like water from a leaky radiator. It seems almost impossible for you to do anything at all.

Fatigue actually suggests two things. First, it is a symptom of lupus. Second, it shows that the disease may be active. When lupus is active, it can cause fatigue (it doesn't matter which particular organs or systems in your body are affected). It's like saying that fatigue is a result of lupus's actively affecting your body.

Although most people think of fatigue as negative, this is not always the case. It can be positive. How? Fatigue is your body's way of telling you that you need rest. If you didn't feel tired, you would push yourself too much! Then you'd certainly feel the effects. So if you feel fatigue, you should listen to your body.

What Causes It?

In a condition such as lupus, fatigue is usually caused by the disease. This is a physical kind of fatigue, and the best way to treat it is to treat the disease that is causing the fatigue. However, this may take some time.

Of course, fatigue can be caused by doing too much! Or it can occur even if you haven't been too active. In this case, the fatigue can be due to other factors such as anemia, medication, or your emotional state.

What if there are times when your fatigue is emotional rather than physical? Is that possible? In other words, you're tired because of the way you feel emotionally, not just because of physical exhaustion. If this is the case, try to determine what emotional reactions are contributing to the fatigue. For example, fatigue could be due to depression, boredom, worry, or just unhappiness. Once you determine what it is that is making you tired, you can work on improving these feelings.

Anti-Tiring Tactics

What's the best way to cope with fatigue? Rest. (Clever!) Allow yourself longer periods of time for sleep at night. In addition, try to arrange for at least one or two rest periods during the day, preferably in the late morning and late afternoon. This may help replenish some of your energy.

Although rest may not make fatigue problems disappear, it can certainly help. If fatigue is a message that your body is unable to do as much as you want it to do, rest is certainly an important way to gain more control. One problem, however, is that *too* much rest can sometimes lead to more fatigue! This can start a vicious cycle.

Fatigue can also be reduced by efficient planning and pacing. Figure out what you have to do. Schedule activities so that you're not doing too many strenuous things in a row. Make sure you intersperse rest periods with any strenuous activities you need to do. And be flexible. You can never be sure when you're going to have energy, or when you're going to feel too fatigued to do anything.

Learn how to pace yourself during your normal routines. Clara Gottaclean was obsessed with the feeling that if she did not do all of her household chores on Monday, the world would fall apart! However, this was more likely to force her to remain in bed on Tuesday and Wednesday. Clara should learn to spread out her chores: do the laundry on Monday, shop on Tuesday, and so on. Be more organized and you may reduce your chances of being fatigued. Reduce the amount of time spent on exercise-related activities. Spread your energy out productively.

You may have to change your general lifestyle in order to maximize your energy level. Know your priorities. Focus on the top priorities while you still have the energy. In this way, if fatigue sets in, it will be the less significant activities that need to be delayed.

Things you used to do that took extended periods of time may have to be shortened or eliminated. If, for example, you were a professional shopper, one who normally spent six hours in the shopping center, you may have to reduce your shopping time. Be careful that you don't fatigue yourself to the extent that you will be bedridden for days!

Other techniques that you have learned in becoming an "efficiency expert," such as reorganizing your house and making things more convenient, will also help you to do more and to feel less fatigued. Don't feel obligated to make all these changes yourself. Getting advice from professionals can help you improve the quality of your day-to-day functioning.

SUN SENSITIVITY

Old Sol can create a lot of problems for people with lupus. It is estimated that about 40 percent of all individuals with lupus experience adverse reactions to the sun. The other 60 percent or more may not need to be as concerned about the material covered in this section, but since lupus varies so much, everyone should keep the discussion of sun sensitivity in mind. What kind of reactions can be experienced? The degree of sensitivity varies from person to person. People with lupus who have unusual reactions to sunlight are said to be photosensitive. Even small amounts of exposure to the sun can aggravate symptoms and make them feel significantly worse.

What Happens?

If you experience photosensitivity, your skin may be affected. This may take the form of redness or a rash, or you may feel a burning sensation. Your skin may itch. Sun exposure not only can cause a skin reaction, but also may result in a major flare, which could affect any part of your body. It may trigger arthritislike joint pains, headaches, or general aches and pains. It may make you very tired or weak. You may experience nausea. Being out in the sun won't offer the health benefits that we were told we would get when we were younger!

During flares, sun sensitivity can increase. The sun may be even more damaging to you at that time. During remissions, sun sensitivity may not be as much of a problem, but be careful: It is certainly very possible for the sun to trigger a flare even when you're in remission. So if you want to stay in remission, do the smart thing (need I say more?).

What Can You Do?

What should you do if you are sun sensitive? First of all, limited exposure to the sun (such as driving children to school, shopping, walking

to and from work, and so on) is usually not dangerous if you prepare yourself adequately. How do you do this?

There are three ways you can protect yourself from the sun: reorganize your activities to have more control of when you're outside, protect yourself with sun preparations, and protect yourself with clothing.

The time you spend outdoors is important. As much as possible, try to avoid being out at all during the strongest hours of sunlight—the hours during the middle of the day. Early morning or late afternoon hours are not as potentially dangerous as the hours during the middle of the day (such as from ten to three). So if you can, try to arrange your schedule so you will be outside during the safer hours. If possible, remain indoors when the sun is at its strongest. In addition, be aware that even if the sun is not shining directly on you (for example, if you are wearing a wide-brimmed hat), reflected sun can also cause problems. Sun can be reflected off pavement, water, sand, snow, glass, and so on. Sun sensitive reactions may occur even in the shade!

Protection from the sun can be improved by using sunscreens or sunblocks. These creams or lotions have numbers on the container indicating how effective they are in blocking out the rays of the sun. The numbers (called sun protection factors, or SPF) range from 1 to 25 and up. The higher the number, the more ultraviolet rays are blocked from the skin. It is suggested that sun sensitive individuals use a sunblock with the highest SPF possible.

Make sure that you wear protective clothing any time you are out in the sun. Long-sleeved shirts, jackets, gloves, and hats can help. You may even want to carry an umbrella to give yourself extra protection from the sun. So what if everybody wonders why you think it's raining! When you are driving in your car, you're not necessarily protected. Do you like to drive with your arm protruding out of the window? If you do, make sure it's protected. Even on a short drive, this exposure may be harmful. Being out for even a short period of time might cause problems, so always protect yourself. Wear sunblock even if you *don't* let your arm hang out. Remember: The sun's rays can penetrate glass!

Physicians have different opinions as to whether everybody with lupus should use sunscreens. Some physicians believe that if you do not experience skin lesions or other specific systemic reactions to the sun, sunscreens are not necessary. However, others feel that even with no lesions, you should use sunblocks to protect yourself from the possibility that a systemic reaction may occur. The general consensus? Since it is easy to get into a normal routine of wearing these lotions whenever you go outside or whenever you have even limited exposure to the sun, use them. Keep them readily accessible in your bathroom, pocketbook, or brief case, so that applying them will become second nature. They're an inexpensive insurance policy against further aggravation and flares.

What if You're Not Sun Sensitive?

If you have not experienced sun sensitivity, you may be reluctant to restrict outdoor activities, especially if this means you can't participate in certain enjoyable activities such as swimming or taking the family to the beach. Although physicians will not say that you can't do these things, be very careful anyway. Don't overdo, because you never know when you may have a sun sensitive reaction, even if you've never had one before. Getting a sunburn, for example, has caused severe reactions in some people who have never had this symptom before.

Is the Sun the Only Villain?

If you are photosensitive, you may be sensitive to more than just the sun. Some individuals with lupus have reported that ultraviolet lights also cause reactions. Those reactions can be very severe, often as uncomfortable as those resulting from sun exposure. Lupus flares can result simply because of exposure to ultraviolet rays in fluorescent lighting.

Therefore, if you are photosensitive, you might want to stop using ultraviolet or fluorescent lighting, and use incandescent lights instead. If you go somewhere where you can't pull out the lighting (imagine going to a friend's house and ripping out all of her fluorescent lights!), you may even want to use sunscreens or sunblocks indoors. A little advance planning can help you feel better.

Summing Up

Don't feel that you should avoid stepping outside, or become obsessed with the idea that you can't expose yourself to the sun. Don't put black tar paper on your windows, or join the Human Owl Society

of America! By preparing for your jaunts outdoors, and by protecting yourself as much as possible, you can minimize any negative effects of being out in the sun. These precautions also apply to people without lupus. Plenty of people who don't have lupus also have to (or want to) be careful in the sun.

NEUROLOGICAL INVOLVEMENT

Neurological problems occur in 50 to 75 percent of individuals with lupus. The statistics may be misleading, however, since something as common as a headache may be considered a type of neurological problem. So don't let the numbers get to you, and keep in mind that this section indicates different possible symptoms. By no means does it imply that you're going to experience them. And if you do, remember that treatment has improved all aspects of lupus, including this one.

Two Types of Neurological Involvement

There are two types of nervous system involvement that may occur in lupus. One is central nervous system involvement, which includes the brain and spinal cord. Problems of central nervous system involvement include focal seizures (trigger activity localized in one specific part of the brain), generalized seizures (trigger activity spread throughout different parts of the brain), and psychotic-type behavior. The other type is peripheral nervous system involvement, which may affect nerves throughout the rest of the body, potentially involving the five senses and movement.

What are some of the specific neurological problems that can occur? In addition to the seizures and psychotic behavior mentioned before, cranial nerve problems may affect movement or the use and function of the eyes. Cranial nerve eye problems range from complete blindness to visual field defects, or double or blurred vision. There may also be problems with eye motion, problems with the pupils of the eyes, or the droopy eyelid syndrome. Nerve damage may result from a restricted or lost blood supply to those nerves, and, on infrequent occasions, may become permanent.

Additional possible neurological problems are tremors (where movements are uncontrolled), weakness (which may exist in arms or legs, or both, on either or both sides of the body), lack of coordination, dizziness, stroke, headaches, and movement or balance problems.

Symptoms involving the central nervous system (called lupus cerebritis) can appear as a neurological problem or as a psychological problem. That doesn't mean people with lupus are flaky, although the anxiety or depression you experience may be related to lupus activity. The confusing thing is that it's sometimes hard to determine the cause of the problem. It is estimated that this occurs in 20 to 50 percent of all people with lupus.

Tests for Neurological Involvement

Among the laboratory tests that are performed to determine if neurological involvement is present and to what extent are the MRI (magnetic resonance imaging), EEG (electroencephalogram), CAT scan, and spinal tap. X-rays may also be used on occasion to see if some kind of neurological damage is involved.

Treatment

Which treatments work best for neurological complications of lupus? It's hard to say, simply because there are so many neurological symptoms that come and go quickly. So it's hard to determine which treatments are effective. However, because in so many cases neurological complications begin while you are not taking any medication or steroids, or when you're on a very low dosage, treatment for neurological problems in lupus primarily involves the use of steroids. Most individuals with neurological involvement improve rapidly after steroid therapy begins or after steroid dosages are increased.

Prognosis

Please don't be alarmed by all of these possible complications. As you know, the prognosis for lupus has improved remarkably over the past several years. Problems resulting from neurological complications of lupus have also been much more controllable recently. So the severity of neurological involvement in lupus has decreased significantly. It is important, however, that these symptoms be recognized if they do come along, so that immediate and accurate treatment can begin.

PERICARDITIS

"You gotta have heart." And you do. You also have a lining around your heart, called the pericardium. If this lining becomes inflamed, the resulting condition is called pericarditis. This symptom is being discussed because one of the most frightening feelings anyone can experience is a tightening, gnawing pain in the chest. "Uh, oh," you may panic, "heart attack!" So it's important to be aware that chest pains are not uncommon in lupus, and one of the causes may be pericarditis.

What Happens?

Inflammation and fluid accumulation in the pericardial sac prevents the heart from moving as freely as it should be able to. As a result, it cannot pump blood as well. When the heart doesn't pump efficiently, two things happen:

1. More blood accumulates in the heart because the heart is less able to send it around the body.
2. Blood supply throughout the body is diminished.

If blood doesn't circulate through the lungs, you may have difficulty breathing since your blood is not able to cleanse the air you breathe by eliminating the carbon dioxide.

A major concern about pericarditis is that if it occurs repeatedly, scar tissue can form in the lining around the heart. This will permanently diminish the heart's ability to beat as efficiently as it used to.

What Can You Do?

Chest pain is the most common symptom of pericarditis. When you inhale, your lungs expand. Because this presses the heart against the chest wall, you'll feel more pain. Try to breathe more shallowly. Smooth but shallow breaths may not hurt as much as deep breaths.

The pain from pericarditis is not as severe when you are sitting up. That's because of the positioning of the different organs when you're in a sitting position. You might want to sit up or bend forward to try to diminish the pain of pericarditis. By the way, this is one way of distinguishing between pericarditis pain and other possible cardiac problems.

Since this symptom is a type of inflammation, other ways of dealing with pericarditis include the same types of medication that are used for other inflammatory symptoms. You guessed it—steroids.

Pericarditis is a major complication. Any symptom that you feel might be evidence of pericarditis should be reported to your physician immediately!

RAYNAUD'S PHENOMENON

Cold hands, warm heart! Have you ever heard that saying before? Unfortunately, it is a painful accuracy for people who have Raynaud's.

Lupus is an inflammatory disease. If the blood vessels are involved, blood circulation may be restricted. In Raynaud's phenomenon, spasms of the small blood vessels severely reduce the supply of blood to the extremities (the hands and feet). Although Raynaud's can be very uncomfortable at times, it is usually mild and rarely results in any permanent damage. Fortunately, Raynaud's phenomenon does not necessarily remain with you forever.

What Happens?

With Raynaud's, some areas of skin (usually your fingers or toes and sometimes even your nose and ears) may change color due to the reduced circulation of blood. If you have Raynaud's, it's unusual to experience the phenomenon in one hand only, although one hand may be affected more than the other.

You may feel a tingling sensation when you are exposed to cold. You may sometimes feel this even when you experience stress. If you have Raynaud's phenomenon, you're probably ultrasensitive to changes in temperature. Your blood vessels are very sensitive to these changes in temperature, and constrict (get smaller in size) very quickly, much more quickly than in a person who doesn't have Raynaud's. All of our blood vessels are passageways designed to allow blood to flow smoothly. The walls of the blood vessels contain muscles. These muscles constrict or relax the passageways, allowing for the movement of blood according to current body conditions. Blood vessel muscles also assist the heart in pumping the blood throughout the body. In Raynaud's, the muscles in the blood vessel walls are so sensitive that they may contract and remain tight for longer periods of time. This reduces, if not totally shuts off, the flow of blood to the extremities. Now you know why you feel the tingling sensations and see the color changes in your extremities.

What kind of color changes will occur as a result of Raynaud's? First, you may notice that your fingers or toes are turning white, especially at the tips. Then you may notice that your extremities are turning blue. Why? The red blood cells trapped in the constricted blood vessels give off their oxygen to the point where they become bluish. When the blood vessels dilate, they fill with fresh, fully oxygenated bright red blood, and so the extremities now look red. So the colors red, white, and blue are common for Raynaud's. Does that mean Raynaud's is a patriotic symptom?

You'll probably notice Raynaud's more frequently during the winter months than in the summer months. However, for some people, being exposed to air conditioning, or even a gust of cool summer air, can bring about a Raynaud's-like response.

What Can You Do?

Try to minimize your exposure to extremely cold or widely varying temperatures. Since stress can cause physiological changes in your blood vessels, try to control stress more efficiently. And, although it goes without saying, smokers should *stop* smoking! But try as you may, it is unlikely that you'll be able to control every possible trigger for Raynaud's phenomenon. So what can you do to feel more comfortable? Keep your hands and feet warm: wear gloves and warm socks. Protect your extremities (sounds like a battle strategy). Dressing warmly is essential, which means that keeping your trunk warm is also important (your body, not your car). Also, you should wear gloves even when you're putting your hands into the freezer compartment of your refrigerator. Even a short exposure to cold can trigger a Raynaud's reaction.

If you're still having trouble, there are many medications that help to dilate the blood vessels. This counteracts the reduced blood flow resulting from Raynaud's. However, these medications do not always work. Different psychological techniques such as relaxation, imagery, or biofeedback may help to improve the flow of blood in your extremities without using drugs.

SJOGREN'S SYNDROME

Do your eyes burn frequently, and not from looking at the sun? Do they feel as though someone dropped Krazy Glue on your eyelids? Do you frequently need liquid to "wet your whistle" even though you're not a camel? If you have experienced any of these or other symptoms of dryness, you may be experiencing the effects of Sjögren's (pronounced *show*-grins) syndrome.

Sjögren's syndrome can be a problem for some people with lupus. It is also known as the "dry eyes, dry mouth" syndrome. Why? In Sjögren's, the autoimmune response of the body destroys the glands that secrete mucus. This can affect, among other things, the production of tears and/or saliva, since both of these secretions are produced in glands.

What Can Be Done?

If your glands' ability to secrete has been impaired by Sjögren's syndrome, treatment is currently unable to restore this function. However, artificial saliva and artificial tears have been scientifically developed to increase comfort for people dealing with this problem. Other medications and treatments are available to deal with the other problems associated with Sjögren's.

KIDNEY PROBLEMS

About half of all individuals with lupus will experience some kidney problems during the course of their illness. Kidney dysfunctions develop gradually over a period of time, ranging from months to even years, and they can be serious.

What Happens?

In lupus, some of the antibodies mix with the substances they are fighting and form immune complexes. These immune complexes remain in the blood until they reach the kidneys. They then become trapped in the kidney's filtering membrane, which normally filters the wastes from the blood. When these complexes accumulate, inflammation occurs. This reduces the filtering processes, sometimes inhibiting them entirely. Waste materials that are normally filtered out of the blood continue to circulate in the blood. This is called uremia. Untreated uremia can result in increasingly dangerous physical and mental problems, in some cases even leading to death. Kidney tissues may scar, further restricting the ability of the kidneys to filter wastes from the blood. When this inflammation and tissue breakdown occurs in the kidneys, the condition is known as lupus nephritis.

Diagnosis

How can you tell if you're having kidney problems? Certain symptoms may suggest it: headache, swelling in different parts of the body (including the arms, the legs, the face, and the area around the eyes or around the abdomen), a decrease in appetite, weakness and fatigue, changes in mental attitude and personality, and seizures. Since so many symptoms of lupus might indicate kidney problems, it's important that kidney functioning be carefully monitored through frequent checkups and tests.

Your physician will check your urine for signs of kidney disease, such as cell casts or increased protein. To do this, he might ask you to collect all your urine for a twenty-four-hour period. He can then assess your kidney filtration rate and function by measuring the relative concentration of certain substances in the urine compared with their concentration in the blood. He'll also see how much protein is excreted in the urine over a full day. Depending on these results, he may recommend that you have a renal biopsy, a procedure in which a thin needle is inserted into the kidney and a tiny piece is removed for tissue study.

What Can You Do?

Certain medications such as prednisone, Imuran, and Cytoxan have been effective in controlling kidney involvement in lupus. The exact drug program has to be individually established, but most cases of lupus nephritis can be helped.

In addition to taking medications, it may be important to reduce salt intake and to work to prevent hypertension. Diuretics may be effective, as well as medications that stabilize the heart and circulation.

Prognosis

Thanks to modern medicine, in most cases, kidney problems need not become life threatening. You are usually able to continue functioning normally. On the other hand, even if kidney dysfunction becomes total and permanent, there are still two possible solutions:

hemodialysis, in which the blood is filtered artificially through a machine, or a kidney transplant. Both of these procedures can be helpful for people with lupus.

Despite the dangers of lupus nephritis, it is at least reassuring to know that advances in medical science have improved the ability to diagnose and treat kidney involvement at virtually every stage.

A PHYSICAL FINALE

This chapter has discussed some of the more common physical symptoms of lupus. Although it is not pleasant to think about your symptoms, you do want to learn how to cope with lupus, right? So you need to know what the possible symptoms of this illness are. But remember: Virtually no one gets all the symptoms, and especially not all of them all at once!

14

Pain

Ouch! (Just getting you ready for this chapter!) Is lupus painful? Are you kidding?! Many individuals with lupus believe that the pain is the hardest thing to deal with.

What can you do about your pain? How can you cope with it? The best way to cope with pain is to get rid of it! To do this, it's first necessary to identify the cause of the pain. Once this is done, treatment can be aimed at eliminating the cause. But there's a problem. In some cases, it may be impossible to do anything about the underlying source of the pain. Since the causes of lupus are still not known, treatment aims to control the symptoms and minimize the pain. So pain itself, rather than the cause of the pain, is the most important concern. What does treatment aim to accomplish then? Relief from pain!

GETTING STARTED

How do you start? First, be aware of your pain. While this may sound strange, you'll learn to recognize whether your pain is something you can (and should) handle yourself, or if it's serious enough to be discussed with your doctor. Remember: If in doubt, check it out. Inform your doctor about the pain. Together you can work out the best ways of dealing with it.

WHEN DOES PAIN OCCUR?

Many factors may contribute to your pain. You'll want to try to control any or all of these factors in order to manage it. Remember that pain can be affected by both psychological and environmental factors. Although pain may initially be physical, emotions can quickly worsen or exacerbate the pain. So pain may result from stress, fatigue, or depression.

Stress causes you to tense your muscles. It may make it more difficult for you to relax, and can increase the degree of pain that you're experiencing. If you're fatigued, you may feel more pain because your tissues and joints aren't getting the rest they need to repair themselves. Depression may cause you to feel more pain because it's on your mind more than it would normally be.

When you're in pain, the degree to which you experience stress, fatigue, or depression may be increased. This can lead to more pain, creating a vicious cycle.

TREATMENT FOR PAIN

There are four traditional categories of therapy for pain control: chemical (using medication), surgical, physical (physical therapy), and psychological. In general, all four therapies work by interrupting the transmission of pain messages before the brain receives and interprets them.

Medical Treatment

Medical treatment for pain generally involves medication. This can effectively control a lot of problems, which can decrease or eliminate the pain. For example, aspirin has been proven effective in controlling minor pain. Steroids are used to control inflammation. When your medication works, joint pain may be controlled. But sometimes discomfort will continue, despite the use of medication. More information about the different medications used in treating lupus will be discussed in the next chapter.

Unfortunately, one of the negative aspects of lupus is that not all pain can be eliminated. For example, dull, throbbing discomfort can continue, despite the use of medication. In extreme cases, surgery may be helpful in treating the cause of pain. But not all conditions lend themselves to surgical treatment. So it may be necessary for you to learn other techniques for dealing with pain.

Nonmedical Techniques

Other than medicine and surgery, what are some ways of obtaining pain relief? Physical therapy techniques, such as using TENS units, heat, cold, and hydrotherapy, and getting a proper balance of rest and exercise, can be used. Some people even look to acupuncture or chiropractic techniques, as well as psychological techniques such as imagery, biofeedback, yoga, hypnosis, and relaxation, to control pain. Last but not least, it's very important to maintain a positive attitude.

You can learn how to employ techniques for controlling pain from physicians, physical therapists, occupational therapists, and mental health professionals (such as psychologists who may specialize in certain pain control techniques). Or you may want to read some of the many books on pain that can be found in bookstores and libraries.

Many techniques for pain control can be applied at home, although in some cases they may achieve greater success in clinics or centers.

Despite the effectiveness of many pain control techniques available today, it's important to consult your physician to make sure that any and all of the techniques are appropriate for you. Make sure that any techniques you're thinking of using are not dangerous for you, considering your condition.

Alleviating the Pain Psychologically

Is pain purely physiological? Rarely, It's usually a combination of physiological and psychological factors. What does this mean? Although your joints may be hurting, it's your *mind* that determines just how much it hurts.

Lisa was limping around her house for hours because of severe joint pain in her ankle. The pain overwhelmed her every time she tried to move faster. Even when she was doing something she enjoyed, her movements were restricted. Suddenly, she heard her 9-year-old son cry out for help. Without a thought about her ankle, she went flying across the room to help him. Her pain couldn't be purely physiological. Yes, Lisa's ankle did hurt, but her mind had probably magnified the amount of pain she felt. When she realized that her son was in trouble, her pain temporarily took on secondary importance.

What does all this mean? If medication or other medical intervention doesn't help alleviate your pain, you can still relieve some (if not all) of it by working on your mind's awareness of it. Read on to find out how you can do this.

Relaxation Techniques

Relaxation can be helpful in controlling pain. Relaxation is the opposite of tension, which can actually increase your pain. Relaxation is also helpful in loosening the muscles that may contribute to your pain. There are a number of different types of relaxation procedures including meditation, autogenic training, hypnosis, and deep breathing procedures.

Let's discuss other psychological techniques to help control pain, such as imagery, biofeedback, and changing your way of thinking.

Imagery

There is a relationship between your mind and the way you feel physically. Much research has proven this. Scientists have also found that bodily functions, previously thought to be totally beyond conscious control (autonomic is the scientific term), can be modified using psychological techniques! One such technique is imagery, or the process of conjuring up pictures or scenes in your mind. In practice, imagery has been beneficial in helping to deal with a host of physiological and psychological problems, including headaches, hypertension, depression, and pain. In many cases, imagery procedures have worked well in combination with prescribed medication for treating illness.

Here's how imagery works. Sit in a comfortable chair or in bed and get into a relaxed position. Lights should be dimmed, and outside sounds or noises minimized, with no interruptions. Breathe smoothly and rhythmically, allowing your body to release tension and to relax. Then imagine a scene of your own choosing, trying to make the image as vivid and real as possible. This scene can be used therapeutically to help you feel better.

Anita was suffering from a sharp pain in her knees. She was instructed to relax and then develop an image of what this joint pain looked like. She imagined it as a very sharp knife jabbed into her knees. Others may feel as if their knees are being hit by a hammer or have dozens of pins stuck into them. Whatever imagery you develop, it should be as vivid and detailed as possible. Anita was then instructed to reverse what was happening in the image: She imagined the knife slowly being removed from the knees, and a soothing cream being applied. Finally, the knife was completely out. She was then able to relax, and her discomfort was eliminated.

There are other images you could use to reduce joint pain. For example, you could imagine oil being squeezed onto the painful joint to allow smoother motion or a soothing lotion being gently massaged on the affected area, or picture yourself taking a warm bath. These images can be used anywhere. (Have you ever taken a bath on a bus?!)

With regular use, they can help you feel better. Imagery is really enhanced by your creativity. A good book on the subject is *In the Mind's Eye* by Arnold Lazarus. See if your public library or local bookstore has it.

Imagery is a key component in hypnosis. Hypnosis may be helpful since it can be quite effective in the area of pain control.

Biofeedback

Biofeedback combines the procedures of relaxation and imagery with the use of measuring instruments—usually electronic ones. These machines let you know what's going on physiologically (giving you feedback) in your body (bio). The devices, which are connected to different parts of your body, provide moment-by-moment information about any changes that are taking place.

Biofeedback can help you learn to control certain automatic body functions by obtaining feedback from certain measurement techniques. You can learn how to voluntarily control internal functions of your body that you may have previously thought were involuntary or uncontrollable. Blood flow or activities of the brain are among your body's automatic functions.

One of the main advantages of biofeedback is that there are usually signals that you can hear or see. Electrodes are either taped to your skin or attached in some other way. They pick up responses that are transmitted to the biofeedback unit as electrical impulses. These impulses are then translated into sounds or lights that you can observe. In this way, you may receive continuous information about body functions such as blood pressure, heart rate, muscle tension, and skin temperature. Using this information, you can develop several different types of imagery so that you can learn how to control your internal responses.

Gayle was experiencing a lot of abdominal pain, so her physician suggested she try biofeedback. A machine measuring muscle tension was attached to her abdomen (in much the same way that electrodes from an EKG machine are connected. There is no pain, and you won't get jolted!). As she attempted to relax her abdominal muscles, the machine gave her instant feedback as to whether she was really relaxing, and to what degree. As she became aware of her lowering tension, she learned what mental images were helping her to relax. She could then continue using these images on her own, without the machine, to help her relax and control some of the pain.

What kinds of biofeedback equipment may be used? Most frequently, machines can be used to measure skin temperature, pulse,
blood pressure, electrical activity resulting from muscular tension, or
electrical activity coming from the brain.

There are some people who wonder whether biofeedback does
anything other than help you to relax your muscles. Further research
is still necessary.

Not much specific research has been done with biofeedback on
people with lupus. However, research has indicated that biofeedback
can teach you how to relax and help you to control pain, warm
hands, and get your muscles to work effectively again. This may be
helpful for individuals with lupus.

Coping Psychologically

There are other factors that can contribute to the intensity (and even
the very existence) of your pain, including your emotional state, the
attention you pay to your pain, and the way the rest of your body
feels. Obviously, as you pinpoint which of these factors do play a
role, you can begin improving the way you cope with pain.

Where do you start? You'll want to do everything you can to decrease fear, stress, tension, and other negative emotional factors. All
of these may make you more aware of your painful physical state.
Anything you can do to relieve anxiety and tension (including psy-
chotherapy, if necessary) should help you to cope better with any
pain.

How do you reduce the amount of attention focused on your pain?
Of course, the more time you have to think about it, the worse it will
seem. So try to divert your attention. Develop other interests that require concentration. You can always come up with pleasant thoughts
or activities that will distract you from painful thoughts. One very
helpful "activity" might be to get involved with a support group for
people living with pain. One such organization is the National
Chronic Pain Outreach. They have many chapters throughout the
country, and more are always forming. It can be comforting to know
that you're not alone in trying to cope with pain. Who knows? You
may even get some great ideas that will help to reduce the pain you
have to live with!

AN UNAGONIZING CONCLUSION

Unfortunately, it is more probable that you will have *some* pain because of lupus. But don't throw in the heating pad! Realize that the pain need not last forever. A lot can be done, both medically and psychologically, to help deal with it.

15

Medication

Other than changes in lifestyle, the main treatment for lupus is the use of medication. Believe it or not, some people welcome drugs as a powerful way to control problems in the body. Others are afraid of their power and of eventually becoming dependent on them. Still others resent the presence of any artificial substances in their bodies. Where do your feelings fit in? Regardless of what your attitudes are toward using medication, your physician has probably made it perfectly clear that you don't have much choice in the matter. Taking medication is not enough—you must take it properly. Otherwise it can be very dangerous. So let's talk about medication, since you must adjust to taking it for lupus.

WHY DRUGS?

Because lupus both creates and is created by physiological problems in your body, medications designed to deal with these problems can be helpful in controlling the disease. There are various kinds of drugs that are very helpful in the treatment of lupus. Some may be used to control flares, reduce inflammation, or suppress symptoms, among other things. Because of the chemical natures of these drugs and the way they may interact with your body, it is extremely important that you follow your doctor's orders in taking the drugs prescribed for you. Do not play with medications that haven't been prescribed for you (or even with the ones that have been prescribed for you, for that matter)!

WHAT TO TAKE

How is it determined which medication is going to be used? In prescribing a drug program, your physician will take into consideration the severity of your lupus at the time and the stage of the illness, as well as the symptoms you're experiencing. Also considered is the amount of pain you're experiencing, what other drugs you're taking, how well you take what you're supposed to take, and your age and overall health, among other factors. But even when all these factors are taken into consideration, doctors are still not sure exactly how certain medication will affect you. So in many cases, trial and error is necessary in order to determine the proper dosage. You may need to try different kinds of medication over long periods of time in order to arrive at the combination that can best help your condition. This may be very frustrating, but the results are worthwhile. Make sure you understand exactly why you're taking medication and what it's supposed to do.

HOW AND WHEN TO TAKE

Besides knowing *what* medication you're taking and *why* you're taking it, you should completely understand *when* and *how* to take it. For example, certain medications should be taken after meals. Others may be taken during a meal. Still others may have to be taken on an empty stomach. Some medication should be taken with water, some with food, and some in other ways.

So far, you know the "what" (which medication you are taking), "why" you are taking it, and "when" and "how" you are to take it. But you also need to know "how much" to take and "how often" to take it. (It seems like "where" to take your medication is really the only thing that's left up to you!) The "how much" and "how often," of course, will be supplied by your physician, but you may still want to understand why it is prescribed this way. Each person has different needs as far as dose and frequency are concerned. What somebody else takes may not necessarily be appropriate for you, even if this person seems to share the same problems. The dosage and the frequency of the medication can also be based on the reaction you have to it, how well it's doing what it's supposed to do, and the severity of the problem that is being treated.

Once you begin taking medication in certain dosages, don't attempt to change these dosages on your own. While some medications may be necessary for only a short time, you may always need other types of medication. However long you must take a medication, recognize that it is being prescribed specifically to help you live as healthy a life as possible. Because of the chemical natures of these drugs and the way they may interact in your body, it's extremely important for you to follow your doctor's orders in taking the drugs prescribed for you. Don't mix drugs without knowing if the combination is safe. Because you may need to take many different pills, it's important that you do not play with your dosage or with the times you take them, or move around the number of pills you take at a particular time. Be sure to follow your doctor's prescription as carefully as possible.

You probably want to take as little medication as possible. Very few physicians will keep you on high doses of any medication unless they feel it's absolutely essential. If you're taking a substantial dose of any drug, then there must be a reason for it. Don't be afraid to ask your doctor about it. Every good doctor will gladly explain your prescribed medication and why you need it. If you're feeling good and think you may not need as much medication as you are taking, consult your physician first. Then you can devise a program for reducing medication together with your physician.

HARMFUL INTERACTIONS

Don't attempt to take any medications other than those prescribed for you. Check with your physician to see if any other medications are appropriate. If you go to other physicians for nonlupus-related problems, there could be a problem if they prescribe medications that absolutely should not be taken with your lupus-prescribed medications. The advantage to having one main physician is obvious. Any other doctor that you may need can then consult your primary physician to make sure treatment strategies will work together, and won't make you worse. Because certain medications are chemically incompatible, you should never mix drugs without knowing if the combination is safe. Don't take the chance. Check it out.

SIDE EFFECTS

Most people with lupus require medication, often for months or years. But that doesn't mean you're thrilled with the idea. Not too many people are. What might bother you? Well, you're probably concerned about what the medication may be doing to your body, or what the side effects may be. This is probably one of the biggest problems concerning medication. Side effects are the "less than pleasant" consequences. They indicate that a drug is interacting with your body in a way other than the way it was intended. Because medication causes chemical changes within the body, side effects may occur whenever medication is taken. Unfortunately, the more powerful the drug, the more potent the side effects. Although no one enjoys the thought of experiencing side effects from a particular medication, at least the side effects show you that the drug is potent. It's working! Hopefully, it will have an impact on the symptoms it is trying to alleviate. So remember that the benefits to your body are usually much more important than any potential side effects. Otherwise, your doctor wouldn't prescribe the medication. Physicians are aware of possible side effects; they won't prescribe any medication that isn't necessary, nor will they prescribe higher dosages than are necessary. If side effects do have a particularly harsh impact on you, then your physician may have to weigh the advantages against the disadvantages. Be aware, however, that the "side effects" of *not* taking prescribed medication may be far more serious than the side effects of taking it!

Minimizing side effects is one reason why it's important to take medication exactly the way it's been prescribed for you. Also, you should report any medication difficulties you experience to your physician. (More about specific side effects will be discussed later in this chapter.)

GETTING DOWN TO SPECIFICS

Let's talk about some of the medications for lupus. The goal? You want to cope with any medicine you have to take as part of your life.

Some of the medications that have been helpful in treating lupus can be divided into six categories:

- Aspirin and aspirin derivatives
- Tylenol and Tylenol-like medications
- Nonsteroidal anti-inflammatory drugs (NSAIDs)
- Antimalarials
- Corticosteroids
- Immunosuppressants

Aspirin and Aspirin Derivatives

Aspirin is part of the family of salicylates, and may be considered one of the most important drugs in the world. That's a pretty bold statement (but true!). It's a relatively safe and effective drug, and, in some ways, a powerhouse. Can aspirin help lupus symptoms? Sure! When your lupus is mild, the first choice of medication frequently is aspirin. Good old aspirin!

Virtually every American family has aspirin in its medicine chest at home. However, if aspirin is going to be part of your treatment for lupus, it should not be taken on a self-prescribed basis. It can be very harmful if not taken carefully. You should use medication for your treatment program only if it is prescribed and supervised by your doctor.

How Does Aspirin Work?

Aspirin can be helpful in reducing the low-grade fevers that frequently occur in lupus. It can also help lessen pain and discomfort. For example, aspirin has been shown to be very helpful in controlling joint pain and joint aches, as well as the chest pain that accompanies both pericarditis and pleuritis. But aspirin is more than just a painkiller. Aspirin can also be helpful in controlling lupus-related inflammation. How does aspirin "know" if it will simply be an analgesic to control pain, or whether it will also act as an anti-inflammatory? The answer is in the dosage! At low dosages, aspirin can help reduce pain. How? It acts on the central nervous system and reduces your ability to feel pain. But if aspirin is going to be effective in reducing inflammation, a higher dosage is needed. Why? Higher levels of aspirin are necessary to block the production of prostaglandins. These are the chemicals that help to trigger and prolong the inflammatory process. Prostaglandins are substances that are released in inflamed areas. These prostaglandins seem to increase the pain you experience because they sensitize nerve endings. By interfering with the production of prostaglandins, aspirin blocks pain and reduces inflammation.

What Dosage?

The correct dosage of aspirin is the one that you can best tolerate. In other words, you should try to keep the dosage of aspirin just below the level at which unpleasant side effects (such as nausea or ringing in the ears) occur.

After taking two aspirin tablets (10 grains), you've usually reached the limit in painkilling ability. If you take more aspirin, you probably won't get much more pain relief. You can usually take aspirin every four hours. Why? Because the effects of aspirin tend to wear off in that time.

On the other hand, if you're going to use aspirin as an anti-inflammatory, you may need a daily dose of ten to twenty 5-grain tablets in order for it to effectively reduce your inflammation. (Make sure your doctor prescribes this amount for inflammation. Don't take it on your own.) You must continue to take this amount every day for weeks at a time if you're going to maximize its effectiveness. Aspirin levels in the body must accumulate and remain high for a period of time before the drug is at its most effective level in treating inflammation. When the aspirin dosage is finally at this level, it must remain there even if you feel better. If you stop taking aspirin or reduce your dosage, the body levels of aspirin will decrease, prostaglandins may increase, and symptoms may return.

Fortunately, aspirin is not an addictive drug. Nor does it seem to lose its effectiveness over time. Although some people find that taking a particular medication often enough leads to a need for more of it to do the same job, it doesn't seem to work that way with aspirin.

Should you take generic aspirin? Most physicians feel that there is nothing wrong with this. As a matter of fact, they may advise you to do so because you will save on costs and still get the same quality. However, if you were doing well on a brand name aspirin, but then began to flare up when you switched to a generic aspirin, it could be that the generic aspirin has less strength and effectiveness than the brand name.

Side Effects

There are possible side effects to taking aspirin. Unfortunately, stomach upset is a common side effect of aspirin. You may also experience nausea or indigestion. Vomiting may occur. Usually, taking aspirin with food, milk, or an antacid may alleviate some of these side effects. Sometimes they can be avoided by using special types of coated aspirin. Liquid aspirin or time-release aspirin may also help to avoid an upset stomach, as may buffered aspirin or aspirin mixed with antacids.

Another side effect from high doses of aspirin is tinnitus, a ringing or buzzing in the ears. Dizziness, slight losses of hearing, or slight changes in vision may also result from high levels of aspirin. Aspirin can also cause a small degree of blood loss from the stomach. While not indicating that an ulcer is present, these surface "erosions" from aspirin can lead to a low red blood cell count (anemia). Black stool may be a sign of blood loss. Sometimes, lightheadedness, increased fatigue, and pallor may indicate that anemia is present. However, if aspirin dosage is lowered or stopped, these side effects practically always go away. But please tell your doctor if any of these symptoms occur.

Any Problems?

There are some people who should not take aspirin. Some asthma sufferers may not be able to tolerate it. Aspirin may cause serious bleeding and, on rare occasions, may even lead to hemorrhaging. People with gastrointestinal problems should always use great caution if told to take aspirin. People who are taking other types of medication, such as blood thinners, may also be advised to avoid aspirin.

People who are allergic to aspirin (although this does not occur very often) must avoid it. There is a difference between side effects and allergies. If you are allergic to aspirin, you must eliminate it from your treatment program; however, if you are experiencing side effects, you may still be able to use it by adjusting the dosage. Symptoms that indicate an allergic reaction include a rash, a runny nose, and wheezing. On the other hand, symptoms such as ringing in the ears, headache, nausea, abdominal pain, and stomach upset are simply side effects.

Why is it so important for you to be able to recognize aspirin's side effects? Like many other people, you may experience side effects from aspirin if your physician has been prescribing it at high doses. If this occurs, talk to your doctor. You may be advised to reduce your dosage slightly in order to determine exactly what the best dosage is for you.

Don't give up on aspirin too quickly. Different brands may reduce the side effects. However, if you experience any of the allergic symptoms mentioned above, these can be more serious. You should then stop taking aspirin and notify your physician immediately.

Tylenol

Another over-the-counter pain reliever is Tylenol. Tylenol, along with other drugs that work like it, such as Datril, Enderin, and Tempra, is useful in countering pain and fever, but doesn't act against inflammation. If you experience stomach upsets or are sensitive to plain aspirin, using these drugs may help.

Nonsteroidal Anti-Inflammatory Drugs (NSAIDs)

Nonsteroidal anti-inflammatory drugs (NSAIDs) are prescribed for lupus because they reduce both inflammation and pain. NSAIDs were cleverly named because they reduce inflammation, but don't contain steroids!

Comparing Aspirin and NSAIDs

How are aspirin and NSAIDs similar? They both are effective in reducing pain and inflammation because of their ability to block the formation of prostaglandins.

However, there are some important differences between aspirin and NSAIDs. Aspirin can be obtained over the counter. On the other hand, most NSAIDs require a doctor's prescription. They usually cost more than aspirin, too. But NSAIDs may be easier to take since you don't have to swallow as many tablets or take them as often as aspirin.

Examples of NSAIDs

There are many different types of NSAIDs. The main difference between them is their chemical molecular structure. (Sorry, further information on this point is slightly beyond the scope of this book!).

Some of the more common NSAIDs include Motrin, Indocin, Tolectin, Nalfon, Naprosyn, and Feldene. Newer NSAIDs are coming out all the time.

Any Problems?

As with aspirin or any of the other medications discussed, NSAIDs do have side effects. Some of the more common ones are stomach pains and cramps, nausea, vomiting, diarrhea, constipation, bleeding from the stomach, and ulcers. Headaches, ringing in the ears, and blurred vision may also occur. Just as certain people may develop aspirin allergies, some may also experience these symptoms when taking NSAIDs. If this occurs, the medication should be stopped and your physician notified immediately.

Antimalarials

Another group of medications that often play a role in treatment programs for lupus is the antimalarials.

How Are They Used?

Antimalarial or quinine-related drugs also are appropriate in treating lupus, primarily to help control the skin lesions that may occur with either discoid or systemic lupus, and to reduce the painful arthritic symptoms of the disease. It is not completely understood how antimalarial drugs work in helping the person with lupus. An added plus for their use is that in some cases, taking antimalarials (such as Plaquenil) enables your physician to reduce the amount of corticosteroids necessary.

The primary antimalarial drug used in the treatment of lupus is Plaquenil. The generic name for Plaquenil is hydroxychloroquine. Most people can tolerate Plaquenil pills. But antimalarials are used less frequently these days, partly because the side effects can be quite serious, and partly because more efficient and less dangerous drugs have been developed.

Side Effects

Many different side effects are possible with the antimalarials. They may be as mild as premature graying of the hair, or as severe as convulsive seizures. Gastrointestinal problems, including severe nausea and vomiting, may occur with antimalarial drugs. Many people have noticed discoloration of patches of skin. However, the most significant problem involves the eyes.

With certain antimalarials such as Plaquenil, changes may occur in the eyes. The most serious side effect of Plaquenil is gradual damage to the retina of the eye, possibly leading to loss of vision in extreme cases. This side effect, fortunately, is uncommon. Because it has been known to occur with the use of some antimalarials, it is very important to see your eye doctor before medication is even started. Antimalarials should be stopped if the slightest change occurs, and you should have your eyes checked regularly (at least once every three months is recommended). In addition, because your eyes will be more sensitive to light when you are taking antimalarials, you should wear protective sunglasses. Wear them in daylight, regardless of whether or not there appears to be strong sun. You may want to wear them under fluorescent lights as well.

Corticosteroids

Many people with lupus are, have been, or may be treated with this category of medication. Corticosteroids (called steroids, for short) have been shown to be effective in treating lupus. However, they must be taken carefully because there can be severe side effects. This is unfortunate because corticosteroids are among the most effective anti-inflammatory drugs known.

Corticosteroids are hormones that are produced by the cortex of the adrenal glands. Nowadays all corticosteroids used in the treatment of disease are produced synthetically.

Steroids are very potent anti-inflammatory drugs. They can quickly reduce pain and inflammation, allergic reactions, asthma attacks, and colitis attacks. There are occasions when steroids are used for short periods of time if an individual is experiencing a severe flare-up of symptoms.

There are many different generic steroids available, including cortisone, prednisone, prednisolone, methylprednisolone, and hydrocortisone, among others. There also are lots of brand names. Each physician usually has a preference. Prednisone is probably the most commonly prescribed steroid.

What Do They Do?

Why are the corticosteroids so helpful? This medication can reduce the inflammation that occurs in lupus, minimizing the damage to internal organs. It is important to control the inflammation that can create so much of the tissue damage in lupus. Since inflammation can also lead to high fevers, steroids are used to reduce inflammation and to keep temperatures in check. Reductions in inflammation can also reduce the pain (such as joint pain) and discomfort you may have with lupus.

So you can see that steroids are extremely important in the treatment of lupus. They are one of the major components of treatment responsible for so much of the dramatic improvement in the prognosis for lupus. Steroids have saved many lives—those of people with lupus, and the lives of people with a number of other serious illnesses or conditions where other treatments were ineffective or unknown.

Your Adrenal Glands May Go On Strike!

All right, you're taking steroids. They're replacing the hormones your adrenals produced. Well, what if your adrenal glands no longer find it necessary to produce their own hormones? They may become less and less active. If you use steroids for a long period of time, your adrenal glands may stop producing altogether. You'll then need the artificial drugs to stay alive. This is one of the main reasons you shouldn't stop your medication suddenly if you are taking steroids. If you do, your body will not be getting any corticosteroids—either natural or artificial. It may take months for your adrenal glands to begin their own natural production of cortisone once again. So a gradual tapering off is the only healthy way to stop taking steroids, but this should be done only when your symptoms seem to be under control (and only under a doctor's supervision). Hopefully, your adrenal glands will increase their production of cortisone as you cut back your medication.

Dosage

What dosage of steroids should you take? Your physician will consider many factors including the severity of your condition and your weight, habits, and age (among other things).

If your lupus is severe or life threatening, extremely high dosages of steroids may be given. If your lupus flare is severe enough to require hospitalization, your doctor may decide to try "pulse therapy," intravenous administration of as much as a gram (1,000 milligrams) a day for three days of prednisolone (the soluble form of prednisone used for intravenous treatment). This is only a short-term measure that often "kicks" your body back into better shape. Then the dosage is rapidly dropped to a more manageable level.

The adrenal-produced hormones primarily help your body to handle sudden, extreme stress. The hormones are secreted mainly when this stress occurs, so if steroids make the glands cut back, artificial drugs must be administered in high dosages at times of extreme physiological stress, such as if you experience a serious injury or if you need surgery. Steroids would be necessary until your adrenal glands have gone back to working full-time.

Under more stable conditions, such as when symptoms are milder, lower dosages will be prescribed. Occasionally, steroids may be prescribed for shorter periods of time, lasting for a few weeks or months.

One Day Yes, One Day No

One strategy that is occasionally used to lessen the chances of unpleasant side effects (usually if you are experiencing mild symptoms of lupus) is to take your medication every other day. In addition, the alternate-day strategy may also lessen the chances of "strike" behavior on the part of the adrenal glands, where they stop producing hormones. However, a problem with this technique is that it is not usually as effective in controlling more active, severe cases of lupus. Don't even consider this technique unless you've discussed it with your physician. Make sure that if the two of you decide to try it, you let your doctor know if your symptoms seem to get worse toward the end of the day that you are off the medication.

How Are Steroids Taken?

Steroids are usually taken orally. They most commonly come in the form of tablets (usually little white or yellow ones). Because they can make your stomach feel like the inside of Mount St. Helens, taking steroids with food can help.

In certain situations (during hospitalization, in preparation for surgery, or during a severe flare) you may receive steroids intravenously (possibly as pulse therapy, which was mentioned earlier), or in the form of injections. Obviously, your physician will advise you of how much medication to take and when to take it. Don't decide on your own to increase or decrease your dosage, or to try alternate-day strategies, because that could be disastrous.

Side Effects

It might seem as if steroids are the answer to your problems if you discount the complications that can occur with the adrenal glands. If they're so great, how come everyone isn't taking them? It isn't that simple.

Although they are extremely important in treating lupus, steroids are not all "peaches and cream"! As with any medication, side effects can be a problem. The potential side effects vary from person to person (just as lupus does!). Your abdomen or cheeks may swell if you have been on steroids for a long time. This is the "moon face" syndrome that is common in individuals taking high dosages of steroids for long periods of time. Not everyone using steroids experiences this swelling. Some don't experience it at all. Others may experience very noticeable changes even with small dosages. This can be depressing, especially if you're sensitive about your looks or weight. Other side effects may include changes in hair growth (slow growth, loss of hair, or increased hair growth on your face and body), an increase in injuries (easier bruising) and slower healing, high blood pressure, a weakening of the bones (osteoporosis), cataracts, an increased chance of infection, depression, and, in some uncommon cases, stomach bleeding (among others).

Another problem is that steroids may mask symptoms, not only ones related to lupus, but also those that may indicate the presence of other chronic or acute conditions. Extensive use of steroids have, on occasion, led to cases of diabetes mellitus, and may cause ulcers or aggravate already-existing ones. (As a note, if you have any ulcer condition or any known active infection, steroids are usually not prescribed.) Your blood pressure may rise from steroid use, so keep monitoring it. Occasionally, emotional problems or other highly individual reactions may occur with steroid use.

Nobody develops all these side effects, and usually they will occur only if you have used steroids for a long period of time. Unfortunately, not too much can be done about these side effects. You'll have to bear with them until steroid dosages can safely be reduced. This takes time.

Summary

What are the most important things to remember about steroids? There are two essential points that you should know if you are taking corticosteroids: (1) because your body's adrenal glands will produce less and less of this hormone, any reduction in your medication should be carried out gradually over a long period of time to allow your normal internal production to begin again; and (2) because of the possibility of your needing greater amounts of corticosteroids during stressful situations, remember to tell any of your physicians, dentists, and other care providers before, during, or after a major stressful situation that higher dosages of the artificial steroids may be necessary.

Steroids are extremely beneficial in many treatment programs for lupus, but they are hardly ideal drugs. Despite their advantages, they are used only in such dosages and for such durations as absolutely necessary.

Immunosuppressants

There are other drugs that physicians have recently begun prescribing for the treatment of lupus. Although still not as prevalent as the drugs discussed above, they should be included in this chapter.

Immunosuppressants (also called cytotoxic or anticancer drugs) are very powerful, but also far from ideal. They are extremely potent, have considerable risks of unpleasant side effects, and, in some cases, can be dangerous. The drugs in this group are often used in individuals who receive organ transplants to prevent rejection of the donor organ. They have been used for many years to treat many different cancers. They have recently been found to be effective in treating some individuals with lupus. Because they are so powerful and potentially dangerous, they are usually used only if other milder drugs are not effective or if the disease appears to be aggressive. Some doctors feel that using immunosuppressants can reduce your need for steroids. The most commonly used immunosuppressants for lupus are Imuran (azathioprine) and Cytoxan.

What Do They Do?

Immunosuppressants are used to reduce the effectiveness of the body's immune system. For example, if Kenny Kidneyfailure needed an organ transplant, his immune system normally would reject the new organ because it was foreign to his body. That wouldn't help poor old Kenny, so he would receive dosages of immunosuppressants designed to decrease the chances that his immune system would reject the transplant. What does Kenny's situation have to do with lupus? The rejection process seems to be very similar to what happens in lupus, where the antibodies are fighting or rejecting healthy cells. So, if these drugs slow down the rejection process, they may reduce the harmful immune system activity that occurs in lupus. They may also fight some of the rebelling white blood cells that are the villains in lupus.

Side Effects

There is an inherent danger in taking immunosuppressants. Since the immune system is being suppressed, it is less able to fight off infection or to protect your body from other possible problems.

There may be a decreased production of cells by the bone marrow. As a result, there could be a drop in the platelet, red blood cell, or white blood cell count. This can significantly lower your body's ability to resist infection. As you know, infections are very common in lupus, and physicians certainly don't want to make you even more vulnerable! Other side effects of immunosuppressants include vomiting, nausea, diarrhea, and heartburn. Skin rashes, easy bruising and bleeding, hair loss, blood in the urine or stool, damage to the lungs, kidneys, and liver, and ulcers can also be a problem. Finally, using immunosuppressive drugs may slightly increase your chances of developing cancer.

In addition, these drugs have been known to interact dangerously with many other drugs. Because of this, some physicians are still very wary about recommending immunosuppressants for persons with lupus. However, other physicians feel they are justified in using immunosuppressants in life-threatening cases when the patient is not responding to steroids.

CAUTIONS

Not all drugs are good for you simply because they are good for others with different health problems. There are certain drugs you should not use because of the possibility of aggravating the symptoms of lupus or causing flares. By working closely with your physician, you will be helping to make sure that all the medications you take are appropriate for you.

There are two types of medications that should *not* be taken: (1) sulfa drugs or drugs that are related to this group, and (2) any drugs that you have had an allergic reaction to in the past. There may be other drugs, such as penicillin or penicillin derivatives, or some of the drugs that are used to control epilepsy, which may present problems (possibly causing what is called "drug-induced" lupus). You've heard it a lot already, but it warrants repeating: Work with your doctor. Question, learn, and help yourself. Check with your physician before taking even the most "innocent" over-the-counter drug. You never know when you might have an allergic reaction. You also have to be careful about any bad mixes. For example, provolone cheese and medication for high blood pressure may not mix! Tranquilizers should never be taken at the same time as alcohol. There are plenty of other such cautions. Please don't hesitate to ask questions. Many of these incompatibilities could have extremely dangerous outcomes, either by making your symptoms worse or by interfering with the desired benefits of the drugs you're taking.

ADDITIONAL MEDICATION 'MINDERS

Once you've begun a medication program, make sure you let your physician know how effective the drugs are in helping you with your condition. Any significant changes in your health, whether good or bad, should be reported to your physician. In this way, your doctor will be best able to decide whether to keep prescribing the medication you're taking.

Keep a list in your wallet of the medications you take. Show the list to your doctor, your pharmacist, or anyone else who needs to know what you're taking. (It makes for entertaining "show and tell" at garden club luncheons!)

You may find that dealing with the same drugstore and pharmacist is very comforting. The more time you spend there, the better the pharmacist will get to know you and your specific case. You'll have somebody else looking out for your welfare in addition to your physician!

It is almost impossible for any physician to keep up with all the thousands of different types of prescription drugs on the market. However, this is the pharmacist's specialty. Frequently, pharmacists know even more than physicians as far as what drugs can go together and what drugs interact dangerously. So it can be very helpful for you to develop a good working relationship with your local pharmacist. Not only will your pharmacist be able to tell you about the medication that has been prescribed for you, but he or she may be able to help you reduce costs. Occasionally, generic products that cost less than their brand name counterparts may be available. However, in some individuals the generic drug will not work as well as the brand name medication. If you have a good relationship with your pharmacist, you will find it a lot easier to get the medication you need.

What happens if you go into a pharmacy with a prescription and the pharmacist suggests substituting another drug (or a generic one) for the medication that was originally prescribed for you? There may be nothing wrong with this, but make sure you consult your physician before making such a substitution. Of course, if your physician prescribes generically, the pharmacist can decide which medication to give.

You may experience certain emotional reactions to taking medication (such as depression or anger). This must be dealt with. (If necessary, look back at the chapters on coping with your emotions.) Remember: If it's really necessary for you to take medication, you might as well let it do what it's supposed to. Accept it and don't let it bother you.

A FINAL COMMENT

This chapter doesn't include all medications used by people with lupus. Instead, it emphasizes the more common ones. But at least this information will give you an idea of what's important to know so you can better deal with taking your medication. So if your doctor prescribes something new, ask about it. Then if your new medication makes you feel better, you'll know why!

16

Weight Changes
and Diet

Food, glorious food! Or is it, "Food, who needs food?" Are you eating less now, and enjoying it less? Some people with lupus experience a reduction in appetite. Along with this may come a desired (or undesired) weight loss. However, not everybody with lupus experiences this. Some people with lupus find they are eating more and, of course, gaining more weight. Steroids may also increase appetite. In addition, steroids used to control the symptoms of lupus may frequently result in a bloating side effect where the face and body swell.

But don't put all of the blame on lupus or your medication! Your weight may increase or decrease, and your appetite may change, but these fluctuations may have nothing to do with lupus. It's easy to blame anything that is happening on lupus. Some people, physicians included, may tend to do this. But perhaps your weight is fluctuating because of binges over the weekend! Maybe you've gone to some food orgies! You may reason that you're probably just retaining water (an abused excuse!). Maybe emotional crises have caused you to overeat. One of the most important things you can do to help stay as healthy as possible is to eat properly and keep your weight at a proper level.

CAN A PARTICULAR DIET HELP LUPUS?

Is there any particular diet that is most appropriate for lupus? The answer is a resounding no! Most persons with lupus do not require special diets; however, it's important to maintain a nutritionally sound and well-balanced diet. A proper diet ensures that we consume all of the necessary vitamins, minerals, and supplements. However, if your doctor feels it would be helpful for you, he may suggest that you try either a reducing diet, a salt-free diet, or a low-protein diet, or a combination of the three. If you have kidney involvement, a salt-free, low-protein diet may be helpful in minimizing water retention.

It is best to avoid fad diets, not because they'll cause lupus flares (they probably won't), but because they're just not nutritionally sound. Your cells need a nutritionally balanced diet to maintain proper growth. Lupus causes your cells enough problems already, without your adding an unbalanced diet to the picture!

If you have lupus, you may occasionally experience certain nutritional deficiencies. During a flare-up, your body may use up certain nutrients at a faster rate than it normally would. This may lead to your feeling more fatigued and tired than usual. Therefore, your physician may suggest that you supplement your diet in order to make up for these deficiencies. However, this does not mean that dietary changes or nutritional supplements are going to eliminate or cure your lupus! So even though lupus is not caused by dietary deficiencies, eating a well-balanced diet is an important part of a complete treatment program.

LET THE EATER BEWARE!

Because diet is on everybody's mind these days, it becomes a very good subject for quacks. You may hear them tell of miracle remedies involving certain types of dietary modifications that are "destined" to cure your physical symptoms. Unfortunately, no diet has yet been invented that can do any such thing.

The types of diets that have been suggested by quacks include ones based on fish, vitamins, fresh fruits and laxatives, or oils, as well as vegetarian diets, low-fat and high-fat diets, low-protein and high-protein diets, and every other combination that you can imagine. But you know by now that there is no such cure for lupus. (There will be more about quackery later.) Even though research is constantly exploring the possible effects of dietary factors on lupus (as well as other diseases), not enough information has yet been obtained to know if certain diets can really help, or how to best implement such a diet, if there is any. (The quacks don't know these things either—they just claim they do. And most people would rather deal with someone who admits we need to know more than with someone who says, "Just listen to me. I have all the answers," even though he doesn't.)

The moral? Eat healthy, eat in moderation, and enjoy!

17

Rest and Exercise

Two important components in your effort to live more comfortably with lupus are rest and exercise.

REST

Rest is important if you have lupus. It gives your joints a chance to "recharge their batteries." It helps you to avoid wearing yourself down. It also helps you to maintain an alert, active state.

Because you have lupus, occasional rest periods may help to keep you as strong as possible for the remainder of the day. However, if you feel very tired too often, your body may be telling you that you need additional rest periods. So pay attention!

Rest is important. But too much rest can be as dangerous as too little rest. Although inflammation may decrease during rest, rest also allows muscles to become weaker and joints to get stiffer. You may feel even more tired. The more rest you get, the more you want, and this creates a vicious cycle.

There are differing opinions regarding how long you should rest. Some people feel you should schedule several five- to fifteen-minute rest periods a day. Others feel you should schedule two thirty- to sixty-minute rest periods each day. There are plenty of other opinions as well. Your physician, along with trial and error, will help you determine which rest periods are most appropriate for you. The amount of rest you'll need will be affected by the severity of your disease, your lifestyle, and other aspects of day-to-day living. For example, if your lupus is in a flare, you may need more bed rest (and less exercise) to give your body extra healing time. Hopefully, this additional rest will reduce your pain and inflammation.

EXERCISE

Exercise may be an important component of your treatment program for lupus. Why? Exercise can build and maintain muscle tone, support and stabilize your joints, reduce fatigue, and maintain or increase mobility. Don't you wish it did all this instantly?

You should try to participate in activities that emphasize good muscle tone, rather than build muscle bulk. For example, walking or swimming are better exercises than weightlifting! It's also a good idea to have a regular exercise program, rather than exercising whenever "the spirit moves you"!

Exercise can help keep your body trim. You'll want to keep your muscles firm, firm, firm—which is better than flab, flab, flab! Exercise can also help your body systems to work efficiently.

But remember the importance of maintaining a proper balance between rest and exercise. Too much exercise may increase the amount of pain and inflammation in your joints, doing more harm than good. This proper balance varies from person to person, and can best be determined by your physician or physical therapist. However, only by trial and error can you really determine whether you are exercising or resting in the proper amounts.

Is Exercise Good Only for Your Body?

Exercise is as important for your state of mind as it is for your body. It is very satisfying because you feel as if you are able to do something. Exercise can build up your self-confidence. Do you no longer feel good about yourself due to your medical condition and the way it has changed your image of your body? Exercise can help. It will restore the confidence you have in your body. Seeing improvement in your performance as a result of exercise can also build up your self-esteem. Exercise clears your mind, keeps you alert, and helps to control some of the unpleasant emotional reactions that may occur from time to time. Exercise can help to control stress, as well as emotions such as depression, anger, fear, and frustration.

In addition to its other benefits, exercise can help you sleep better so you'll feel better the next day. And unless you exercise alone, you'll enjoy some healthy social interactions—always good for the mind (as well as the body)!

Getting Started

The kinds of exercise you do will depend on a number of factors, including the severity of your pain and inflammation, your overall physical condition, and the joints affected.

If your medical condition has kept you from being active, be prepared for a little frustration. When you first begin to exercise again, *wow*, will you be out of shape! That's not a put-down. Your muscles will need time to regain their strength. So any kind of exercise that you do should be implemented gradually. The longer it's been since you've done any exercising, the slower your return should be. And again, to benefit most from an exercise program, you have to do it regularly.

Exercising Caution

Not every exercise is appropriate (or even safe) for every person. So make sure you have your doctor's approval before doing any exercise. Then start building up your exercise ability gradually. Don't exceed the moderation that's required.

You'll want to learn the difference between muscle soreness (which may be a normal response to exercise) and acute joint pain (which is a result of that particular exercise, and may mean that you're either overdoing it or participating in an exercise that's a no-no). The old adage, "No pain, no gain," is not necessarily accurate if you have lupus. What you really want to do is enough exercise so that your muscles feel good each day. You're trying to improve both tone and strength.

Be careful to avoid exercising certain parts of your body for too long. If you exercise an inflamed joint, the inflammation may temporarily worsen. Therefore, although exercise doesn't necessarily have to stop if your joints are inflamed, it should focus either on joints that aren't affected, or very carefully (and minimally) on joints that are.

Categories of Exercise

What are you trying to accomplish through exercise? The answer to this question usually determines what category the exercise fits in. In other words, exercises can be classified as range of motion, stretching, muscle strengthening, or endurance (or functional) exercises.

Range of Motion

A joint's normal movements (in different directions) fall into the category "range of motion." Has lupus reduced the range of motion possible in any of your joints? If so, exercise may be able to stop that reduction. Just as importantly, it may be able to gradually increase the range of motion that is possible.

Range of motion exercises stretch joints in various directions by manipulating the muscles attached to them. Range of motion exercises may be very helpful in preventing loss of motion, restoring lost movement, and reducing stiffness. They also help you to maintain normal movement in your joints.

Strengthening Exercises

Some exercises are important because they build up strength in the muscles or other tissues that support the joints and keep them stable. These exercises also help maintain the strength that you already have.

There are two types of strengthening (or muscle-tightening) exercises that may be helpful for you: isometric and resistive. Isometric exercises are strengthening exercises that do not involve any movement within the joints. In these exercises you strongly tighten the muscle but do not move the joint. As a result, strength can be improved without further stressing the joints. Resistive exercises actively move the joint against a resistance, such as a weight, or against other objects. Because there is less chance of stressing an already fragile joint, isometric exercises are usually considered safer than resistive exercises.

Positioning or Stretching Exercises

Positioning exercises can also be helpful, especially for the hips, knees, hands, shoulders, and back. By stretching your body into certain positions, you may be able to help keep these joints limber. Examples of positioning exercises include reaching a high spot on the door and stretching out on your bed.

You can do stretching exercises to relieve any stiffness or tightness in the muscles or tendons surrounding a joint. If pain immobilizes a joint, the muscles controlling that joint are not doing anything. This disuse will adversely affect the muscle, causing such problems as spasms, cramps, and decreased flexibility. Stretching exercises can help get rid of these problems.

Endurance Exercises

Endurance exercises are also referred to as aerobic exercises. These are less beneficial for specific joints, but are more helpful for overall fitness. They are usually a good complement to range of motion and strengthening exercises. Examples of exercises for endurance are walking, swimming, and bicycling. Endurance exercises build up heart and lung strength. They can also reduce chronic fatigue and improve overall physical fitness.

Active Versus Passive Exercises

You can also categorize an exercise as either active or passive. If you're moving your body without anybody else helping you, you're doing active exercises. If you're moving it and someone is helping you, these are active assistive exercises. If you "relax" while a physical therapist, family member, or friend moves your joints (for example, if you're in a severe flare), then you're doing passive exercises.

Guidelines for Exercise Benefits

To be sure you derive the most benefits from your exercise program, use the following guidelines:

- Don't feel that you have to wait until you feel better before starting an exercise program. Starting sooner may even help you to feel better more quickly. Just make sure you get professional advice and supervision.
- Try to build up your tolerance to exercises slowly. You can improve the way your joints and muscles function by regularly increasing the amount of exercise you do. It is important that you do this gradually. Too rapid an increase, or too intense an exercise program, may only increase the pain that you're experiencing. It

may also damage the very joint that you want to protect and improve.

- If you experience a lot of pain or inflammation in your joints, exercise must be done with much more caution. Isometric exercises may be helpful. Very gentle range of motion exercises may also be suggested.
- Anticipate minor discomfort from exercising. Remember, you're moving joints that may not want to be moved! Bending a joint and stretching the surrounding muscles, tendons, and ligaments may cause some pain. Some professionals recommend pushing a joint just a little beyond the level at which pain first occurs, because this may help to increase joint mobility. But if you experience too much discomfort or pain, or if it lasts for a long time (an hour is too long), cut back. It probably indicates that you're overdoing!
- Aim to do as much exercise as possible on your own, although you should initially get help in selecting your exercises from either your physician or a physical therapist.
- Don't compare your exercise program to somebody else's. You wouldn't compare your doses or types of medication to somebody else's, would you?
- If you decide to join a gym for your exercise program, beware of instructors who tell you they know "just what will make you feel better." They may know very little, if anything, about lupus. A better course of action would be to come in with suggestions for exercise from your physician or physical therapist, and simply ask the instructor to see that you're following your exercise program correctly.

A Final Calisthenic

Exercise can be either extremely valuable or extremely harmful (or anywhere in between!) depending on the care you use in approaching this activity. Because every person with lupus is different, there is no one set of exercises that is recommended for everybody. But everybody can benefit from something! Don't just jump in feet first. Use your head. Speak with your physician or physical therapist, start exercising slowly, build up your stamina, and enjoy your exercise program as you feel better.

18

Activities

What to do, and what not to do—this is what you need to decide. Sure you have lupus, but what does this mean in terms of the basic activities in your life? What *can* you do and what *can't* you do? Even if you feel wonderful, you'll probably want to curtail any vigorous activities. You don't want to put any strain on your body. In fact, you may not even have the strength!

Each person is different. The kinds of things you did before being diagnosed with lupus can influence what you can or want to do now. Your current physical condition is also a determining factor. If you're in the middle of a flare, for example, you may not want to expend a lot of energy until your doctor has given you the green light (or even a cautious yellow) to resume activity. So let's discuss some of the more important types of activities that people participate in.

WORKING

Working can be very important for you. Besides being a primary source of income (can't overlook that!), working will make you feel like your life is proceeding as usual. You may be concerned (an understatement!) that your lupus might interfere with your ability to work. This may threaten your financial security.

Even though you have lupus, you'll probably want to do as much of what you used to do as possible. Are you afraid that you'll feel like less of a person if you have to stop working? Work is important. It helps you to feel independent, gives you a sense of self-fulfillment, and provides financial security. You also will benefit from social interaction with colleagues.

Many people question whether they should work. If you want to, and you need to, and you can, then you should! You may have to make some modifications because you don't want to chance running yourself down.

Where to Work

Five basic points may help you when you are resuming your old job or starting a new one. First of all, ask yourself if you feel comfortable doing the job. Do you feel physically and emotionally capable? Is it something you want to do? Your condition may have made you more aware of your mortality. As a result, you might decide to start doing something you really want to do! Second, if you had been working before and had to take a leave of absence because of a flare, will your employer take you back? Or will a new employer hire you, given your present physical condition? Should you even say anything about it? (More about this in a later chapter.) A third very important matter is whether your colleagues will accept you. This, of course, does not mean that they will even notice your condition. Fourth, will your condition affect your attendance at work or your punctuality? If so, will this cause any difficulties on the job? A fifth factor that may relate to your choice of employment is the amount of stress involved. Stress is certainly a factor you'll want to minimize, since it can exacerbate your physical condition. You may decide to change jobs if you recognize that your previous job was too stressful.

Stamina Shortage

Lupus may cause you to experience fatigue, depression, and adjustment problems. This may affect your work productivity, especially if your treatment is not controlling your symptoms as well as you'd like it to. Your productiveness may decrease, you may be absent more often, and your value to the company may decrease. You simply may not feel physically able to work. You may get tired easily, and feel that you just don't have the stamina necessary to complete your job satisfactorily. You may need to be off your feet more, or you may have been told not to walk up and down stairs. If your employer is aware of any of these problems, you may be afraid that your job will be in jeopardy.

What can you do? Build up your stamina slowly. Don't expect too much at once. Pacing yourself is probably the most important thing you can do. Take frequent rest breaks to "recharge your batteries." If you're not sure how much you can do, do what you can and let your body be your guide. Regulating the amount of medication you take for pain is very important in this respect. If you take too much, you won't be aware that you are overdoing it because your pain will be suppressed.

Bending the Rules

Employers are not required by law to make any special provisions for you because you have lupus. You still have to do what you're supposed to do. However, if you're an important employee, your company will probably want to retain your services. You may be able to continue working at a particular job with only a few modifications (such as changing your chair, desk, or location, or a few of the activities you used to do). Changing your hours may also be helpful.

You may be uncomfortable about approaching your employer to find out if these changes can be made. It may bother you to seek special treatment on your job, but this is something you may have to do. If you are a valued employee, these changes may be small in comparison to the problems your company might face if they had to hire a new employee to replace you.

You may fear that you'll have difficulty with other employees if you receive special treatment. This may not be true at all, but your anticipation or apprehension of this happening may cause problems.

Changing Jobs

Don't stay at a job if it's not right for you. Consider transferring to another one or getting additional training to move into a new job. In some cases, individuals with certain job experiences and backgrounds are unable to work in jobs for which they were trained because of their new condition. For example, Lenny, a 39-year-old father of two, had been working in construction. But doctors felt he shouldn't continue this type of work because it was too strenuous for him. Lenny became very depressed. He didn't know what else he could do. He shut down emotionally in order to avoid facing the prospect of not being able to work. He was even afraid that he didn't have the ability to go out and get new training.

How do you deal with this situation? One way might be to check with the Office of Vocational Rehabilitation (OVR), a service provided by the government. The Office of Vocational Rehabilitation can be a very important resource in helping you get back to work. You'll find office locations throughout your state. Counselors in these offices will work with you to determine exactly what your aptitude is for different jobs. OVR will then provide you with training and support to help you obtain employment in those fields. In addition, they also provide transportation, counseling, placement, and even equipment (when necessary). If you've been having difficulty getting a new job and are not sure how to proceed, calling your local Office of Vocational Rehabilitation may be an excellent way to begin. If you need help in finding jobs that are appropriate for you, you may want to check with the State Employment Services. These services are available free of charge and have specialists that can help you find jobs that are suitable for your needs.

Is Working Your Only Option?

What are the advantages of working? Some of the benefits are satisfaction, productivity, money, and pride. But what if you can't work? Or what if you're between jobs? A paying job is not the only type of satisfying work. There are plenty of other meaningful, productive activities that can be done voluntarily. Check with nonprofit organizations, hospitals, schools, senior citizen centers, and the like. They can always use some extra help. You'll feel good about yourself, too. Volunteers can also work with religious, political, or charitable organizations.

What if you just don't want to work? Some individuals with lupus are happy about not being able to work. But don't use your condition as an excuse for not working. This may indicate that something else is bothering you. You may want to explore this further.

SCHOOL

The problems you will face while going to school are similar to those experienced by people with lupus who work. Attendance may decrease because of times when you just don't feel up to going. You may be concerned about going to school because of physical restrictions or the reduced number of activities that you can participate in.

A child with lupus may be concerned about the comments of other students while in school. Teachers should be informed so that they are made aware of these potential problems.

THERAPEUTIC RECREATION

People with lupus may still be able to participate in a number of different types of activity including boating, skating, golf, tennis, and dancing. Whether or not you do depends on your condition. If you try an activity without experiencing excessive fatigue, pain, swelling, or other problems, you're probably O.K. On the other hand, there may be times when you think that you can't do something because of your condition. However, if your doctor approves, at least you'll know that you can try. It's up to you and your doctor to decide which activities are best for you.

Why is it so helpful to participate in activities that you enjoy? One reason is that they can help improve your ability to take care of yourself. They can also help promote and maintain your participation in the normal activities of daily living. They can certainly enhance your social life and improve your spirits as well.

ACTIVITIES OF DAILY LIVING

Among the things you'll do each day are the normal, routine tasks known as the activities of daily living (ADL). But there's a problem. The restrictions you're experiencing from lupus may limit these activities. This can be frustrating. Why? Probably because prior to being diagnosed, you may have taken such simple tasks for granted. The way you're feeling now, however, may make you depressed and upset, rather than enthusiastic about trying to conquer the problem.

What if you can't do what you want to do? You may not want to ask for help. You may feel that it takes away some of your dignity. This can make you very uncomfortable. However, the future can be brighter! In a very short period of time, you can reorganize your lifestyle, your house, and your daily activities, in a way that can reduce your difficulties and salvage a lot of your dignity. Remember: Not all people with lupus experience these problems. (And if you do, doesn't it make sense to see what you can do to improve the situation?)

Modifying your lifestyle or your home is not the same as giving in to lupus; rather, these changes will help you learn how to live most effectively and cope most successfully with your condition.

Easing the Load

Your goal is to make daily living as easy as possible. Why? One of the most important components in your treatment program for lupus is energy conservation. So you'll want to eliminate those activities that aren't necessary and simplify those that are! Conserving your energy can be very important in helping you to avoid much of the excessive fatigue that can be a negative factor in living with lupus.

In many cases, problems with daily living can be conquered without professional help. It can be very satisfying for you to develop your own solutions to these problems. This can be one of the most important ways of coping with lupus. Of course, any questions you have can be bounced off physicians, physical therapists, or other therapists.

Start by trying to evaluate everything you do on a day-to-day basis and seeing how you can make every single thing you do easier. Realistically, you know you cannot eliminate all of the activities that you need to do around your home. However, what's wrong with finding easier ways of doing them? Are you being lazy? Of course not. You are simply recognizing that every bit of energy you save from one activity will give you more energy to do something else.

Any specific suggestions? There are lots of things you can do to help yourself with daily living. For example, you may want to reorganize your home and your habits in such a way that makes movement easier and puts things within easy reach. You can replace small handles on drawers with bigger ones. You can lubricate drawers so that they open and close more easily. You can wear clothing that is easier to get on and off. There are a number of different types of gadgets that may make life easier for you.

You'll also want to learn how to moderate your activities. Plan them out carefully and pace yourself. One thing you may find helpful is to chart out your activities, including required activities as well as social and leisure activities. This may help you to become better organized so that you can pace yourself more effectively.

Try to plan activities in advance so you can figure out exactly how you're going to do them, what equipment you're going to need, and how much time you can spend doing them in between rest periods. With planning, you may reduce the amount of strain, both physical and emotional, that you experience, and keep yourself from getting overtired.

Try to reduce the amount of energy you expend in performing any activities. If necessary, modify the method that you use. Eliminate any unnecessary activity. Rest intermittently, frequently, and whenever needed. You'll then be able to do more of what you want or need to do. And you'll accomplish it in a healthier way.

Any activities that cause you pain should be modified as much as possible. And you certainly don't want to do anything that causes severe pain, even if it is very short-lived. If you've already reduced a task to the bare minimum, and absolutely can't do anything more about it, put a limit on how much pain you're going to let yourself endure. An ache that lasts five to ten minutes may be bearable if it is not severe, but severe pain may be a problem.

A FINAL EXERTION

Keeping active is a very important part of coping with lupus. You want to feel productive and enjoy life. You don't want to let lupus confine you to your closet. So don't let it. Do what you physically can, but *do. . . .*

19

Financial Problems

Having lupus can be a pain in the pocketbook! Any chronic illness can be expensive, and lupus is no exception. However, the cost of living with lupus that is the most devastating is the human cost: the pain and suffering that must be endured.

Why are the financial costs so high? The cost of treatment, doctor's visits, and other medical costs, as well as the cost of medication, hospitalization (if needed), and laboratory tests, all add up. In addition, money is lost from the number of work days that are missed because of symptoms. The cost varies considerably for each person with lupus. It doesn't take long for financial security to drain into a financial problem.

INSURANCE CAN BE AN ASSURANCE

Fortunately, some people can have some of their costs defrayed by insurance. Insurance coverage is essential. For individuals with lupus, certain costs may be reimbursable by third-party payments. Insurance companies do cover a number of our medical costs. But what happens if you run out of money or insurance, or if your coverage is not good enough? Because you have a chronic illness, you may have more difficulty getting either life or health insurance. Speak to a reputable insurance agent and find out exactly what you are entitled to. Also speak with a social worker to learn what your community offers in the way of aid.

DECREASED WORK, INCREASED COSTS AT HOME

Financial problems arise from lost earnings or income. You may not be able to work at all, or perhaps you can hold down only a part-time job. Your condition may affect your ability to work. This may cause problems with your job. So it's possible that your "employability" will be reduced because of your lupus.

Lupus can also be costly because of changes at home. You may need to have other people help you, or you may need to make renovations in your home. You may need help around the house, such as a baby sitter or a cleaning person. All of these things cost money, adding to your financial burden. As your medical costs rise, your budget will become tighter and tighter. If costs continue to skyrocket, you may feel as if you're being strangled!

CAN ANYTHING HELP?

Although lupus can be an expensive disease, it need not be alarmingly so if you're careful. If you take proper care of yourself and follow your treatment program correctly, hopefully you'll be able to prevent the more serious (and expensive) problems that can occur.

The use of generic medication can save you money. Generic medication is sold by its chemical name rather than by a more common brand name. Ask your physician if it's acceptable to take generic medication. (Remember, not all generics work as well as brand name medication.)

If medical costs are overwhelming you, consider attending a clinic. Because clinics usually operate on a sliding-scale fee schedule, you may be able to get quality medical care at a reduced cost. In some cases, you may even see the same physician you'd normally see, since many physicians graciously donate their time to clinics.

If you are experiencing financial problems, you may want to check with either the Lupus Foundation or the Department of Social Services. They may be able to provide you with information, resources, and, in some cases, emergency assistance. They can tell you which benefits you may be qualified for and how to apply for them.

So before you do anything, talk to people. Find out what others have done. How do you find them? Ask your physician or nurse for suggestions, or contact your local chapter of the Lupus Foundation for ideas. Speak to others in similar situations to find out how they handle their money problems. Even though you may initially be embarrassed to bring up the subject, the common bond that exists among people with lupus tends to smooth this over rather quickly. You'll be glad you brought it up!

UNCLE SAM TO THE RESCUE

Some government insurance programs may be very important sources of financial support. You may be covered (at least to some degree) by Medicare, where eligibility is determined by age, chronic disability, or both; Medicaid, where benefits vary from state to state; or Social Security Disability Insurance. Let's discuss these different government programs, what they do, and how you can participate (if you're eligible).

Social Security (Disability)

If you are unable to work because of your lupus, you may be eligible for disability benefits. However, you may experience all kinds of legal problems because of the many different definitions of disability.

The Social Security Disability Program is a federal government program. It is administered and run by the Social Security Administration. The money that funds the Social Security Benefit Plan comes from workers and their employers. Therefore, in order to receive benefits, you must meet certain qualifications. First, you must have worked long enough, earning an appropriate number of "credits," and second, you must have worked recently enough. The time requirements are determined by the age at which you became disabled. In other words, if Olivia Outofdough wanted to receive disability benefits, the age at which she became disabled would determine how many credits she would need to qualify, and how recently these credits must have been earned. For further information, or for help with your particular situation, call your local Social Security office. Its personnel can check your employment records and tell you your status.

Benefits are available from the Social Security Disability Program to those of you who fit into one or more of the following four categories:

1. Individuals under the age of 65 who were disabled (and their families).
2. Single individuals under the age of 22 who were disabled before that age and are still disabled.
3. Widows who are disabled.

4. Widowers who are disabled and also dependent.

There are also other specific cases that may entitle you to benefits.

There is one very rigid rule that the Social Security Administration enforces in order for benefits to be approved. This guideline is: "The physical or mental impairment must prevent you from doing any substantial, gainful work, and is expected to last (or has lasted) for at least twelve months, or is expected to result in death." In other words, it is expected that your disability prevents you from doing any meaningful work. This must be the case if you are applying for disability benefits.

Once you meet the eligibility requirements for disability benefits, does that mean that cash will start pouring in? Not so fast! There are still other steps that you have to go through. You'll have to provide the names and addresses of people involved in treating you, including physicians, hospitals, and clinics. Medical records must be provided, substantiating the dates and treatments prescribed. This information will be evaluated by a Social Security team (including a physician), and additional tests may be required to support your claim.

The medical requirement for disability from lupus includes:

1. A positive LE prep test, and a positive finding on the test for antinuclear antibodies.
2. Frequent manifestations of the following types of problems related to lupus: cardiac problems, kidney problems, central nervous system involvement, gastrointestinal problems, or pulmonary problems.

The word "frequent" in requirement 2 does not necessarily mean every week! Meeting this requirement depends on who is evaluating your claim. "Frequency" may depend on either the symptom or its intensity, as well as the interpretation of the investigators. If a serious symptom occurs only once every six months or so, it still may satisfy the requirements because of its severity.

Supplemental Security Income (SSI)

Once you apply for Social Security benefits, you also become eligible for Supplemental Security Income. This leads to eligibility for Medicaid. The Supplementary Security Income Program is also run by the Social Security Administration, which operates the Social Security Benefit Program. However, whereas Social Security benefits come from workers and their employers, SSI comes from a general treasury fund.

SSI benefits are available to individuals 65 and over, the blind, and the disabled. Disabled individuals who receive SSI benefits must fulfill the same definitions of disability that are used for Social Security benefits.

Medicaid

Medicaid is the more commonly used term for Medical Assistance. Benefits are provided automatically for anyone who qualifies for Supplemental Security Income. Medicaid will cover virtually any medical-related expense, as long as you go to a professional who is a "participant provider." This provider is then directly reimbursed by the state for the service provided to you.

Medicaid applies if you are 65 or over and are receiving Social Security, or if you are under 65 and have met the Social Security requirements for disability. In addition, Medicaid is provided to families on welfare.

Medicare

Medicare is another part of the Social Security Administration. There are two components to the Medicare Program. The medical insurance component helps you to pay for physicians' services and outpatient services, including physical therapy and speech pathology. The hospital insurance component covers inpatient care and nursing care within a facility.

Medicare benefits are limited and rigidly evaluated. They are applied only to charges that are deemed reasonable and necessary in treating your disease. In order to be eligible for Medicare benefits, you must have received disability checks for at least two consecutive years. This applies only if you are under the age of 65, since Medicare benefits are provided to anyone 65 years of age or older. Another acceptable criterion for receiving Medicare benefits is if you have permanent kidney failure that requires dialysis or a kidney transplant. This is not a frequent occurrence from lupus.

WHAT SHOULD YOU DO?

To determine whether any of these programs are applicable to you, contact your local Social Security office. In addition, consult your physician or your local support groups. These sources should provide you with valuable information that will assist you in determining which programs can help you. But beware. These programs are strict. The government, it seems, is more eager to reject your claim than to accept it. You can appeal if your application is rejected, but this becomes even more aggravating. Want some advice? Talk to people who have been through it, such as members of your local support groups. Contact your local lupus organization. The Lupus Foundation of America has put out a comprehensive guide book to disability rights and programs. This book should be available from the national chapter (see address in the appendix) or from your local chapter. Fight for your rights—and for your dollars.

$UMMING UP

Although lupus can be costly, there's still hope. More and more people are learning about it, and about its costly impact. Hopefully, the variety of insurance coverages available to you will increase, more provisions will be made for meeting your expenses, and requirements and application procedures will become more humane.

20

Traveling

Ellen was a 42-year-old executive. One of the reasons she always enjoyed working hard at her job was that it provided her with an income sufficient to take her family on luxurious annual vacations. She and her family would spend many happy weeks in many different parts of the world. However, since she was diagnosed with lupus, Ellen had not taken any trips at all. Why? You see, Ellen was afraid that her disease would interfere with her sightseeing plans, so she didn't want to go at all. Need it be this way? Definitcly not. Very few restrictions need to be placed on your travel plans. As a matter of fact, you can probably go just about anywhere!

If you think you might like to travel, discuss it with your physician first. Chances are that if you're able to get around your own neighborhood without assistance, you can probably handle traveling with confidence. If you do have difficulty getting around, you'll want to be more selective about where you go. (And obviously, if you're in the middle of a flare, this might not be the best time to travel. Want a tip? Always take out trip cancellation insurance, especially if you stand to lose a lot of money because of last-minute, nonrefundable cancellations.) If getting around is a problem, you may opt to use wheelchairs to reduce fatigue as well as to increase the distance you can travel. Although wheelchairs are a good idea for some people, others are afraid of being seen in a wheelchair, or are even more afraid that once they use them, they'll be stuck in them forever. Neither of these fears is valid, but both can interfere with happy travel plans. Work on them.

Do all individuals with lupus avoid traveling? No. Some don't travel simply because they feel it's too expensive. This may have nothing to do with lupus. But plenty of others do travel, whether their trips are short or long. Some travel simply to prove to themselves that they can. This doesn't mean that there are no fears attached. Many want to prove to themselves that they can do it—that traveling, one of life's pleasures, is possible for them, too. As with any other aspect of living with your lupus, planning ahead and taking the proper precautions can allow you to travel with a free mind (although not with free airfare!). How should you plan ahead for a vacation? Let's explore some of the things you should do.

When making hotel reservations or other accommodations, make sure that they fit your needs. You'll want to know where you can get proper medical care if necessary. So prepare for this. Write out a list of clinics, hospitals, and physicians in the different parts of the world where you may be traveling. In addition, find out if there is a local chapter of the Lupus Foundation at your destination. This can be very comforting to know.

TAKING MEDICATION AND OTHER SUPPLIES

Running out of medication or other supplies may be one of your biggest concerns about traveling. There are two things you can do. First, have extra medication and supplies packed in case any unexpected situations arise. Second, ask your physician to write up extra prescriptions to take with you. At least you'll be prepared if you need more. You may also want to ask if you can keep your doctor "on call," so you can contact him or her in an emergency. If you're going to a foreign country, you may want the prescription translated into the language of that country in case the pharmacist has difficulty understanding English. If you are flying (in a plane!), you should carry medication and other necessary supplies with you. Do not pack all supplies in your luggage. Why? If your luggage ends up in Birmingham when you're flying to Los Angeles, you don't want to be left without what you need. Besides, if for any reason you need a pill during the flight, it would be rather inconsiderate of you to ask the flight attendant to climb down into the baggage hold to get it!

IDENTIFY YOURSELF!

It's always a good idea to travel with complete identification, not just for your luggage but for yourself. The Medic Alert bracelet is accepted worldwide as identification of a person with a medical problem. In addition, make sure your wallet contains an identification card with complete details about your condition, the type of medication you need, and any other pertinent information. Again, if you're going to a foreign country, you might make sure that this information is translated into the language of that country. What if foreign languages were never your forte? Try checking with a teacher of that particular foreign language in a local school. Check with the airline that travels to that country. Representatives who speak the language would probably be willing to translate for you. As a last resort, you may want to check with the foreign embassy of that particular country. This may take a little extra time, but your mind will be more at ease when you do travel.

AIRPLANE ANTICS

Let's say your vacation is set, you're flying to Paradise, and you're now making final preparations before leaving for the airport. Any special considerations? You bet!

If you have any physical restrictions, discuss these in advance, either with an airline representative or with your travel agent. Airlines frequently have special services for individuals with restricted mobility. For example, you may be able to board early, select your seat in advance, have wheelchair access to and from the gate, and have special meals, if necessary. If you have your own wheelchair and you plan on traveling with it, check with an airline representative to find out what regulations apply.

TO SUN, PERHAPS TO FLARE

You know if you're photosensitive or not. So you know whether this needs to be taken into consideration when you decide on your destination. But even if you can't sit in the sun, this doesn't mean you can't go to a sunny place! Just use proper protection, as we discussed in Chapter 13, "Physical Changes." Yes, you may wish you could join your family at the beach. But at least you can join your family in all other activities, if you're not fit for the beach. And after all, who wants to look like a prune from too much sun?

EATING ABROAD

Eating and drinking in a foreign country occasionally can cause problems for any traveler. Therefore, you really have to be on your guard and be aware of potential problems. Unless you've been assured that it's O.K., don't drink tap water or even water in thermoses provided by hotels. Avoid fruits and vegetables that may have been washed before being served. Avoid any other foods that include water in their preparation. Even something as simple as brushing your teeth can make you wish you were back home in bed. You've heard of Montezuma's revenge? Well, Montezuma has traveled to many parts of the world! The best way to conquer the water problem is to use pure, sterilized, or distilled water. Some hotels will provide water purifiers so that you can take water from the tap, process it, and then be able to use it safely.

It is not always safe to drink even typical American soft drinks when abroad. The name of the soft drink may be American, and the packaging may look the same as it does in the United States, but that doesn't mean that it has been made in the United States. If the drink was manufactured or even bottled locally, you still run some risks.

In addition to being cautious of the liquids you drink, you should also discriminate between foods. Any foods you do eat should be well cooked and properly prepared. Avoid foods that do not look or smell the way you'd expect them to. It's better to be safe and hungry than full and uncomfortable.

If you do want to eat fruits or veggies, peel them carefully, throw away the peels, and wash them with purified water. If any food has a broken skin or looks damaged, throw it away. You're usually better off not eating any foods that haven't been cooked. Canned baby foods that are available in large markets can be good dietary supplements (remember, you did like them once!). Here is a disappointing thought, however. Pastries, especially those made with cream, can be dangerous (and not just to your waistline)! If they're not prepared and stored properly, bacteria can grow on them. If you want to eat meat, be very careful about where you eat and what you choose to eat. American laws are very strict about the inspection of meats served to the public. Laws may not be as strict or may even be nonexistent in other countries. Therefore, you run the risk of eating improperly cooked meats, meats that have not been prepared appropriately, and so on. Use good judgment. You may ask, "Why can't I eat this when the people who live here eat it all the time?" Don't be jealous. You don't know if that's true. You don't know if they eat these foods or if they avoid them, too. Or maybe natives are used to these foods and their lead-lined stomachs can handle foods that your stomach can't. Perhaps hundreds of natives are home in bed with food poisoning! At any rate, be sure to protect yourself.

Are you beginning to think that because there is so much to be afraid of, you won't be able to enjoy your vacation? Don't feel that way. Just remember—you're not going on vacation merely to eat. (If you are, don't go someplace where food is such a problem!) Instead, try to emphasize the other, more enjoyable aspects of your trip. Adequate preparation and total awareness are easy to achieve and will certainly help to make your trip an enjoyable one.

CRUISES

More and more cruise ships have special accommodations for people with physical restrictions. Some have rooms specifically designed for individuals with limited mobility. Ramps may have been built and doorways widened for greater accessibility on some ships. If you're planning on taking a cruise, make sure that you know what ports of call the ship will be stopping at. In certain Caribbean ports, for example, the ship does not dock at the pier. Rather, it drops anchor away from the pier, and small boats are used to get you ashore. This may be more difficult for you to handle if you have any physical restrictions. Again, if you're taking your own wheelchair, be sure to find out what regulations may apply.

TRAIN TRAVEL

Quite a variety of passenger trains exists throughout the country and abroad. Some trains are very accessible for individuals with disabilities. Others are not as accommodating. If you're thinking of traveling by train, speak with a railroad representative or your travel agent before making a final decision.

BUS TRAVEL

Bus travel is becoming easier for people with disabilities. Even if you need a wheelchair, it can probably be stowed, and somebody can help you to get on and off the bus.

A FINAL CONFIRMATION

Remember, not everyone is like Ellen. Many individuals with lupus feel absolutely no reluctance to travel anywhere. If you haven't traveled recently, you may want to build up your confidence by taking short trips first. Taking a three-month trip around the world might be a bit much! Even an overnight trip might be traumatic. Start with a couple of day trips, then take weekend trips, and work your way up to short-distance, week-long excursions. Expanding your travel activities slowly is a good way to develop your confidence. There are special travel agencies for people with disabilities. Look in your local Yellow Pages.

A lot of information has been provided here—mostly precautionary, but nevertheless realistic and sensible. You may need extra time to prepare for your vacation (more time than the "average" traveler). However, with this extra preparation you should be able to enjoy a wonderful vacation, just as anybody else would. Don't forget to send me a postcard!

21

Quackery

Elaine was frustrated. She had been taking medication for months to relieve her lupus symptoms. Although her pain had somewhat diminished, she still wasn't able to do what she wanted to do. Doctors constantly told her there was nothing else that could be done for her at this point. Therefore, her eyes lit up when she read an advertisement for a "cure" for joint pain. Without thinking twice, she wrote out a check for $39.95 and mailed it to the "pharmaceutical" company which described a particular nutritional supplement that guaranteed it would "relieve your joint pain symptoms in less than thirty days, or your money back."

Three weeks later she received the small vial of bitter-tasting pills. When she had finished all the pills after thirty days, not only did she realize that her physical pain had remained the same (fortunately, she had continued to follow the treatment program prescribed by her physician), but she also had the added mental anguish of knowing that she had been duped!

When you're dealing with something as long-lasting and uncomfortable as lupus, it's important that your illness be treated properly. But what if you become impatient with your treatment? What if it doesn't seem to bring about results as quickly as you'd like? You may become tempted if somebody suggests a particular technique or item that is the "latest miracle cure"! This is the lure of "quackery."

WHAT IS QUACKERY?

Quack remedies are treatments that are fraudulent because they do not have a scientific basis. They do not have a sufficient amount of scientific evidence to prove their effectiveness. In other words, there is no reason to believe that they will work and, in all probability, no real evidence that they do! These quack techniques are usually promoted to the public in an extravagant way. Your vulnerability is what's at stake, and whoever is hawking the technique is trying to take advantage of your condition.

Where did the term "quack" come from? In the seventeenth century, the term "quacksalver" was used to describe a charlatan who bragged that certain products had magic curative powers. These phonies didn't know anything about medicine or about their patients. The term "quack" is an abbreviation for quacksalver.

Not all quacks are blatantly cruel people. Some people believe that their techniques work and think that they can actually help you. In some cases, remedies may be advocated even by doctors, and it may be hard to differentiate or distinguish these from legitimate treatments. However, you still want to be wary. You don't want to be the unsuccessful guinea pig who eventually learns that such techniques are worthless!

HOW MUCH DOES QUACKERY COST?

Unfortunately, billions of dollars are spent each year on quack remedies and devices. This has become a very serious problem (except for the quack!). And here's another mind-boggler: For every dollar that is spent on legitimate and appropriate scientific treatment for lupus, more than twenty-five dollars is spent on quack remedies, phony pain relievers, and inappropriate cures!

WHO'S SUSCEPTIBLE TO QUACKERY?

If you've been experiencing never-ending pain, increasing disability, and problems with your joints, you may be vulnerable to the suggestions of a quack. If you feel that your physician isn't helping you as much as you'd like, you might find yourself susceptible to the promises of a quack.

Don't be ashamed to admit that you've been approached by, or even considered buying from, a quack. Virtually anybody who has been affected by a chronic medical problem has been taken in at least once. (I won't ask if you're one of them—your sheepish grin is answer enough!) Consider yourself lucky, however, if you recognized your mistake early enough and were able to avoid being taken for another ride.

So why do so many people fall victims to quackery? The quack promises a quick, easy cure for a long-term problem. You already know that traditional treatment programs for lupus do not work overnight! In some cases, especially when you're most vulnerable, it's simply too hard to pass up! You may figure, "What do I have to lose?" (A lot!)

HOW CAN QUACKERY HURT YOU?

What will you lose if you try a quack remedy? Besides money, there are a number of things that you may lose. You may also lose patience, confidence, dignity, courage, and, in certain extreme cases, life!

Money can be a problem. Although it may cost you only a few dollars for a book or copper bracelet, it can get more expensive when fraudulent programs of injections or spa treatments are involved. These may cost thousands of dollars. Remember, a quack isn't in business for ego building or gratification. A quack does it for the money!

Quackery may convince you to forego standard medical treatment. If this happens, you won't derive appropriate benefits from whatever medical treatment can be helpful to you. There is also the danger that the quack approach may cause additional damage. This may occur if the quack treatment conceals symptoms that need prompt, proper treatment.

Trying a quack approach may be not only financially draining, but also psychologically draining. If you build up your hopes that something is going to work, then when it doesn't, you feel even worse than you did before. This disillusionment can certainly undermine your courage and determination to live with your condition. Your patience may be sorely tested. You may find it even more difficult to participate in an appropriate treatment program.

It can be terrible to lose your dignity. You may feel that you've been ripped off, or that somebody has taken advantage of you. Your integrity and pride have been damaged. Don't continue to feel this way. Write off what you've done as experience. Accept the fact that you were deceived and move on to more appropriate treatment.

EXAMPLES OF QUACKERY

The different types of quack techniques may be divided into three categories: drugs, diets, and devices. What are some examples of miracle cures with little validity? Consider some of the following:

- *Drugs*. Indian medicines, vitamin injections, iodine.
- *Diets*. Immunized "milk," alfalfa seeds, crow meat, gelatin, seaweed, worms, yogurt, mineral waters, fasting, eating only uncooked foods, eating only cooked foods.
- *Devices*. Copper bracelets, electric belts, magic horse collars, magnetic devices, zinc disks, teeth extractions, mistletoe, polyvinyl clothing, special underwear, sulfur baths, applications of a hot poker, electric shocks, sitting for prolonged periods in abandoned uranium mines.

A Little More Detail, Please?

Many of the quack remedies are based on changes in diet. Keep in mind that extensive research has indicated that other than eating to keep healthy, no major dietary changes have either prevented or exacerbated lupus.

Whenever you read of a "diet to cure lupus," you should be a little skeptical. Why? The key word is "cure." At the present time, lupus cannot be cured. In some cases, these diets may be more damaging because they may not provide you with the nutrients or fluids you need for a balanced, healthy diet. Research hasn't shown any indication that a specialized diet can play a role in helping lupus. Therefore, you should be wary of an individual who says that a particular ingredient will make your lupus symptoms go away.

Venoms are often advocated as ways to cure the arthritis symptoms of lupus. Venoms from animals or insects such as snakes, ants, or bees have been touted as being miracle cures. What's the danger? What if you're allergic to these venoms? You might experience reactions that are more serious than even lupus itself!

Some people believe that wearing copper bracelets can be helpful because the chemical nature of the copper can alleviate a deficiency within the body. The answer to this is simple: If you enjoy wearing a copper bracelet, and you feel it's attractive and adds to your looks, fine. But don't expect it to result in significant changes in your lupus.

Certain clinics may also fall under the quack category if they promise miraculous cures costing a mere several thousand dollars. It is true that in these days you get what you pay for. This may cause the unwary individual to believe that paying a lot of money increases the likelihood of success. Promoters are aware of this, and will milk you for as much as they can.

PROTECT YOURSELF!

With all of the unproven methods and quack remedies promoted in magazines, in books, and through different individuals, how can you tell which are real and which aren't? It may be hard to decide if a remedy is really quackery, especially if, while using a quack remedy, you go into remission! But you have to ask yourself whether it was really the quack remedy that was responsible for this or if it could have been a "placebo effect," in which your strong belief in what you were taking or doing helped to produce the desired effect. Might this have happened anyway due to your regular treatment program? Perhaps this was a spontaneous remission. What if the disease returns later in full force? If you're convinced that the quack treatment did cause the remission, dependence on it may prove extremely dangerous.

How can you protect yourself from quacks and their remedies? Before trying anything, investigate it carefully. Be suspicious. Be cautious. Speak to your own physician. You should also be aware of other individuals who may claim to be physicians to try to convince you that they have a cure for lupus. Check the validity of a "treatment" with the Lupus Foundation, the Food and Drug Administration, or the National Institutes of Health.

Sometimes your physician may not be able to tell you whether a particular remedy is valid. In many cases, physicians are so busy that they may not be aware of or understand the technique that the quack is trying to push. This may confirm, in your mind, what the quack has been saying all along—that the medical profession disregards the needs of the person with lupus and doesn't have time to investigate all the possibilities. This may bother you, and may make you more vulnerable to what the quack is saying. Quacks know this. That's why they're using this argument in the first place! Don't let them cause you to doubt your physician. There may still be good reason to reject the idea that the quack is trying to sell you on.

Although some quack remedies may seem harmless, they can still hurt you if they keep you from following an appropriate treatment program for lupus. Keep that in mind. Try not to let anyone convince you that you should no longer follow an appropriate treatment. If you have questions about whether your doctor is prescribing the treatment that's best for you, it's better to get a second opinion from another physician than from a quack!

BEWARE OF THE "RED FLAGS"!

What should you beware of? Any of the following could be a give-away that the remedy is quackery:

- Beware of any procedure that promises quick, easy relief of pain.
- Beware of any treatment program that advocates a special diet or nutritional approach as the answer to lupus.
- Beware of any secret formulas, devices, or programs that will "cure" lupus. At the present time, there is no cure for lupus. If any kind of miraculous discovery were made, you would be sure to learn about it in the newspaper, on the evening news, or from some other reputable source.
- Beware of quacks who claim that their cure or remedy is exclusive or secret. You might ask them why honest people would keep their cure a secret when it could help so many people. Or ask them why you didn't hear about it through a more appropriate channel! Scientists who are a legitimate part of the medical world do not keep such discoveries exclusive or secret.
- Beware of any technique that has no scientific proof of its safety or effectiveness. Keep in mind that the promoter probably hasn't had any kind of clinical trials to test the method.
- Beware of anything that is advocated in a rag magazine or tabloid, through a mail promotion, or by somebody whom you meet in a store or at a meeting.
- Beware of any advertisements that offer testimonials or case histories of individuals who are satisfied with a particular program or approach. If somebody indeed finds an answer to helping people with lupus, it will not be necessary to advertise.
- Beware of people who claim that they know exactly what you're going through and what symptoms you're experiencing, and then explain how they're going to help cleanse your body of any poisons it may contain.
- Beware of anybody who attacks the standard medical treatment of lupus or who states that appropriate medications are unnecessary because they're damaging and dangerous. Quacks may claim that medical professionals are deliberately withholding treatment approaches that can be more helpful. Some quacks may accuse the medical profession of trying to interfere with attempts to get their remedy approved. Frequently, these attacks will be launched

toward the Lupus Foundation, the Food and Drug Administration, and even the American Medical Association.

- Beware of the efforts of friends and family to persuade you to try a quack approach. Their suggestions may be harder to resist than advice given by strangers. Your family and friends really want you to feel better. They don't like to see you suffer and are eager to find some kind of solution to your problem. This may make *them* ripe and vulnerable to a quack's suggestions, which they'll then pressure you to try. Now not only will you have to resist the remedy, but you may also have to conquer the guilt that may arise if you don't try the "cure" they found. ("Why won't you try this, dear? Don't you want to help yourself?")

THE FINAL QUACK UP

It's always important to do the best you can to help yourself. You definitely want to feel better, and you want treatment to do the best it can to help you. You don't want to waste time, money, or psychological energy on quack remedies. Always aim to do the best you can to help yourself, but use appropriate means!

PART IV
Interacting With Other People

22

Coping With Others—
An Introduction

You do not live your life alone (unless you're reading this book on a deserted island in the Pacific). You interact with many people every day. So you'll certainly want to be able to deal with any difficulties in interpersonal relationships. For example, what will others think about your lupus? How will they react? Will they ask questions? What kinds of answers will they be receptive to and what kinds will they reject? These are some of the questions that may bother you. Since you'll probably be with other people during a good part of your waking hours, it makes sense to be aware of how lupus can affect these relationships. Obviously, different problems can exist in different relationships. But before we begin discussing each type of relationship specifically, there are a few general points to be made.

DO UNTO OTHERS . . .

When you interact with others, you don't want to become too wrapped up in your own feelings. If you disregard the feelings of others, you'll also prevent them from getting close to you. Consider how others feel, just as you'd like them to consider your feelings. What does this mean? You're not the only one who has to cope with lupus. Important people in your life are also having a hard time, simply because you mean a lot to them. Remember that. Some people tend to feel that their problems don't affect anyone else. You might think, "How can they feel upset? It's happening to *me*!" But is that fair? Take your family, for example. A problem for you is also a problem for them. Of course, it may be affecting you differently. You may be the one experiencing the restrictions and the physical changes, as well as the apprehensions and the anxieties, but your condition still affects those who care about you. They don't like to see you suffer. If you remember this, you'll be better able to cope with these important people and with your condition.

YOU CAN'T CHANGE OTHERS

Do you feel that if you try hard enough, you can change the attitudes, feelings, or behaviors of others? It doesn't happen that way. Whether they accept your lupus or deny that you have any problem at all, you can't change them. You can change only yourself. Spend more time working on yourself, and worry less about others. They may change, but it will more likely be a result of the changes they see in you. Help yourself. Be your own best friend.

LOOK THROUGH THE EYES OF OTHERS

If you have an argument with someone, you may believe that you're right and the other person is wrong. In this case, nothing will be resolved. Take a moment and look at the situation through the eyes of the other person. What does he or she see? What might the other point of view be? Trying to see the other perspective will help you to better understand the problem.

If you look at the problem only through your own eyes, someone else's behavior may drive you crazy. Looking through the eyes of others can help you better understand them and improve your relationship with them. If you try to have a discussion with them, you will also be able to explain how *you* feel.

PRIDE, YES! REVENGE, NO!

Revenge! There are times when you might think, "I only wish that _____ could know what it's like to live with lupus for an hour, a day, or a week, so that he/she could understand what I've been going through." But you know this isn't realistic, and you can't sit around waiting for it to happen. Besides, afterward you might not be too pleased with yourself for having such vengeful thoughts. So what should you do? Take pride in yourself. Concentrate on doing what's best for *you*. If you have to be a little more self-centered and a little less concerned about what other people think, just accept this as one more way of coping with your condition.

A LITTLE SELFISHNESS IS O.K.

What happens if you're feeling rotten, but others want you to keep doing more and more? In the past, you may have had trouble saying no, either because you'd feel guilty or because you didn't want to disappoint someone or hurt his or her feelings. But now you must curtail your generosity because it can hurt you. Frequently, you may have to give the appearance of being selfish. But don't take this negatively. As long as you don't abuse it, this selfishness can be positive for you. Do for yourself; think of yourself. You're Number One, and that's the way it must be. If you take care of yourself, then you will be in the best possible shape to deal with others. The reverse does not hold true. If you are best for others, you may not be best for yourself.

BRING ON THE WORLD

Now that we've started with some general ideas, let's see how lupus can affect the many different relationships you have with people. Of course, not every chapter will apply to you. You may either read the chapters that are appropriate for you, or read them all to see how different kinds of problems exist in any relationship.

23

Your Family

Because blood is thicker than water, your family can be a critical factor in your successful adjustment to having lupus. Why? You're probably with your family more than with anyone else. If you get along well with members of your family, you'll have a solid foundation from which to move toward a triumphant adjustment to your condition.

There are various types of problems that may pop up with different members of your family, so let's discuss how to cope with each specific member of the family.

COPING WITH YOUR SPOUSE

Of course, lupus has a definite effect on your marriage. But this doesn't mean that problems can't be resolved. Through better communication, understanding, and counseling (if necessary), there are very few problems that can't be worked out. Let's discuss some of the ways in which a marriage may feel the impact of lupus.

Social Life Changes

Have you had to cut back on your social activities because of restrictions caused by lupus? You may have to curtail some of the activities that you used to enjoy with your spouse. You may not be able to do as much. These changes can be hard to bear, especially if you both had active social lives before the onset of your condition. Because your spouse does not have lupus, he or she may feel anger, frustration, or helplessness. If your social life is still on hold even after your condition has stabilized, you'll have to ask yourself if this is due to certain fears or apprehensions. If so, refer to other appropriate chapters (such as Chapter 7, "Fears and Anxieties") for suggestions and support.

If Family Responsibilities Must Change . . .

Lupus may create the need for temporary or permanent changes in each family member's responsibilities. This can surely be another potential source of friction between you and your spouse, especially when your spouse receives a heavy share of the load. Reassigning chores to different members of the family can be very difficult for all.

Sheila, a 36-year-old mother of three, returned from a doctor's visit and immediately called a family powwow. She told her husband that because she did not receive a good medical report, he would have to take over all of the household chores, including all the cooking and cleaning (even washing the windows). Her two older children would have to do all of the grocery shopping and would have to take turns helping their younger brother with his homework, bathing, and other daily routines.

Despite the fact that Sheila's family loved her and was concerned about her health, they were all understandably upset, especially her husband. Since he had difficulty boiling water, he certainly wasn't happy about his new assignment. The two older children may also have a hard time dealing with their new responsibilities. How can you adjust your routine as smoothly as possible? Make changes gradually. Being able to afford household help would make things easier for the whole family, of course. But regardless of whether you have paid help, try to avoid overwhelming your spouse. Be realistic in your expectations.

How else can you help your spouse to adjust to greater burdens? Make sure free time is still available for the pleasures of life. It's only when the new responsibilities seem to be all consuming that serious problems occur. Look at any lifestyle changes through the eyes of your spouse. Consider how you'd feel if the situation were reversed. Think how upsetting it would be if you no longer had time for things you enjoyed because of added responsibilities and pressures. Discuss the situation reasonably, and be gentle.

Denial

What should you do if your spouse simply won't accept the fact that you have lupus? You might hear, "Oh, come on, you look fine. What are you complaining about?" Your spouse's disbelief may be tough to swallow. You can try to educate your spouse, but don't go overboard. Constantly badgering about all of the things that have changed because of your lupus certainly won't convince someone who has apparently been denying its very existence. Your spouse will not accept your condition until he or she is ready to do so. Concentrate on your own feelings. Others' feelings may change, but slowly.

In Sickness and in Health? Sorry!

Unfortunately, some marriages have ended because of chronic illness. The restrictions of lupus can drive wedges into what may have previously been good marriages. Former feelings of closeness and intimacy may be replaced by the unwelcome feelings of coldness and distance. Some spouses have so much difficulty accepting changes in appearance and behavior that the "magic" seems to be washed right out of the marriage. But it may not be all your spouse's fault. You may be so apprehensive that you can't enjoy your relationship. Your sensitivity may cause you to be less patient. So marital breakups do occur. But realize that about 50 percent of all marriages end in divorce anyway, even when lupus is not involved!

Statistics aside, what do you do if your spouse is frightened and "wants out"? Your spouse's fear, your own condition, and your fears of abandonment all combine to create a horrible package of anxiety, depression, hopelessness, and panic. This package isn't one you can (or should) handle alone, and at this point, you probably won't want to talk to your spouse. You may find communication with your spouse either nonexistent or counterproductive. Get some help. Seeking the aid of a professional or an objective outsider may help to smooth over some of the rough edges. If possible, include your mate. But once again, don't force the issue. It's more important for you, at least, to get some counseling. If your marriage does end, outside support will help you to accept and cope with life without your spouse.

What About Money?

Lupus can present added money problems, especially for your spouse. If you are the breadwinner, your spouse may fear the unpleasant role of becoming more responsible for financial aspects of family management. If your spouse is the major income producer, pressure from the added costs of treatment and medication may be tough. Both you and your spouse will worry about whether all obligations can be met (and whether they can continue to be met). Money concerns are frequently a major source of friction in any marriage. Your medical bills will compound the problem. Sit down, talk it over, and be realistic. Although new strains may arise, these things frequently have a way of working themselves out. Be patient, be communicative, and be positive.

Is Sex Affected?

Another important area in which lupus may affect a marital relationship concerns sex. Chapter 27, "Sex and Lupus," provides more information on this important subject.

A Marital (Con) Summation

Coping with your spouse while you have lupus can be extremely difficult and, occasionally, impossible. Any marriage has its ups and downs, its problems that have to be worked out. Having lupus makes relationships more vulnerable to crises and arguments. Working through lupus-related problems requires much more attention to your spouse's feelings and needs. But it's worth it. If problem spots can be smoothed out, your spouse can be your best ally in helping you adjust to your condition.

COPING WITH CHILDREN

Children need a lot of attention, help, and love from their parents. Lupus can surely be frustrating for everyone if you're unable to provide as much for them as you'd like. You can't do as much or help them as much. This does not mean that you don't love them or that you're not a good parent. Because each person lives differently with lupus, there's no way of predicting how much it will affect you physically (or even emotionally). It may be hard to acknowledge your shortcomings as a parent. But think about your children. How much do they know about your condition? How hard is it for them to deal with it? Let's see how you can help them.

How Do You Explain Lupus to Your Children?

The younger the child, the less of an explanation he or she will need. Anything that you tell a youngster will have to be explained simply. With very young children, you might just say, "I don't feel well and I can't do this. I'd like to, but I can't." Unless you're severely affected, you may not have to say much of anything.

With older children, explanations can be more detailed. Encourage their questions. Sherry Lynn, aged 10, knew her mother had lupus. But her mother couldn't understand why she rarely asked any questions about it. Was she keeping unhappy thoughts inside, or had she just accepted it and didn't feel it was necessary to ask anything? Remember: If your children really don't want to ask you anything, they won't. But let them know that they can if they want to. Upsetting thoughts can be even more destructive if kept inside.

The questions of older children will probably be more direct and more specific. Resulting discussions, if handled properly, will be helpful for your children, and you will enjoy them. You'll also enjoy the comforting feelings of closeness that can result.

Fielding Children's Questions

How do you answer your child's questions? That depends on the age of your child and how detailed your child wants your answer to be. The best advice is to provide direct answers to specific questions. Don't go into detail unless your child asks for more information.

Think, for example, about parents talking with their children about sex. Because of the delicate nature of the subject, and the discomfort or anxiety of the parent, more information than necessary is usually given. Have you heard the anecdote about the very young child who walked up to his mother and asked, "Mommy, where did I come from?" The mother started to tremble because this was the first time she had heard such a question from her child, and she wasn't prepared to answer it. After thinking for a moment, she nervously explained the various parts of the female anatomy and how the sexual act resulted in conception. She told how this ultimately led to the birth of the child. When she finished after about fifteen minutes, she breathed a sigh of relief and expectantly waited for her child's reaction. The child responded, "But Mommy, I didn't want to know all that. I just wanted to know what hospital I was born in!"

The message in this anecdote is clear. Try to determine exactly what your child wants to know. Some children may not even know what answers they are looking for. So just start answering and then ask if that's what they wanted to know. Continue from there.

Be careful not to frighten your child. Children have great imaginations. You don't want your answers to get blown out of proportion. You want your child to continue to talk to you about your condition. If you show that you accept lupus (as much as you can) and the way it affects you, and even welcome questions about it, this will greatly benefit your relationship with your child.

"Will You Die?"

This is an inevitable question. Whenever a child knows that a parent has a serious medical problem, he or she may worry. It may be frightening for your child to see you unable to get out of bed in the morning. You'll have to handle this very carefully. Children become petrified thinking about the death of a parent. They don't understand what you're going through and they will certainly be afraid. Reassure them that you're not going to die. Although these may seem like empty words, that's what they need to hear.

Although lupus is not considered a fatal disease, it may not be enough for you to tell your child that you will not die, especially if you're not sure yourself. (Children are very perceptive; they'll recognize your fears.) It might be a good idea, therefore, for you to speak to a professional (your physician or your child's pediatrician, for example) and to include him or her in the discussion.

Spending Time Together

One of the hardest parts of coping with lupus is handling the disappointment of your children when you can't do all that they'd like you to do with them. You want to be a good parent. But what does that entail? Most parents believe that they must spend lots of time with their children by making themselves available to take the children places and by doing things with them. If they don't do this, parents may feel guilty. But lupus can be restrictive and may prevent you from doing a lot of what you'd like to do. You have no choice. How do you solve this dilemma? How do you explain to your child that you can't take him or her somewhere, or that you can't do what you had promised? Children don't want to understand when they're upset. Making deals can help. Explain to your children that you're not available as much as you'd like to be. Come to an agreement with them about some enjoyable activity you can do together when you're feeling better. This arrangement will show your children that you're aware of their unhappiness and want to help.

Try to spend *quality* time with your children—special time when you really share feelings and activities. You shouldn't be as concerned about the *quantity* of time—the number of minutes or hours—you spend with them. If your time together is precious, then this is much more important than the amount of time you share. Your children will do just fine. Talking with your children and being open with them will also help them better handle your lupus.

COPING WITH ADOLESCENTS

Coping with adolescents can be very different from coping with children. Because adolescents are older and can read more complex material, they can read most of what has been written for adults. They can ask questions if anything they read is too complicated. However, the main difficulty in coping with adolescents is recognizing their special needs.

The Declaration of Independence

It is during adolescence that teenagers begin to assert their independence. Look out, world! The future generation is coming! Adolescents want to start moving away from the family setting and its responsibilities. Under normal circumstances, this can create problems in many homes. Your lupus can cause even more problems. Why? Because of your condition, your adolescent may have to help out more than usual with daily routines and chores. At the same time, the adolescent wants to do less and be away more. What a bummer!

For example, 15-year-old Douglas feels guilty about not helping out more at home, but feels that giving in is a sign of weakness (heaven forbid!). These mixed feelings cause Douglas a lot of anguish, which of course he doesn't want to discuss with his parents. The need to escape seems even greater. So, dear parent, imagine how helpful it can be for you to be aware of your adolescent's feelings. Take the initiative and offer a reasonable compromise. Just showing that you understand will help. Maybe things won't seem so hopeless to the adolescent, after all.

The Need for Friends

Adolescents are usually less interested in spending time with family members, and more interested in being with friends. It may be easier for your teenager to deal with your lupus if his or her friends spend little time at your house—that way, your adolescent need not explain your condition. Even if your teenager's friends don't know about your condition, your adolescent may be much more sensitive to the situation. Does this sound strange? Most adolescents want to impress their friends. Somehow, having a parent who has trouble walking doesn't quite "fit the bill." Of course, there are some adolescents who are more mature and open about it. The extent of their love for their parent and a sound family relationship minimize the problem. They may sometimes end relationships with those friends who cannot understand the situation. Unfortunately, this is not often the case.

Another problem for your adolescent is transportation (that means you!). Many adolescents count on their parents to drive them to friends' houses, parties, meetings, and so on. But you may not be available (or able) to chauffeur your teenager around as much. As a result, you may feel guilty because you believe you're not being a good parent. Your teenager, thinking less of you and more of himself or herself, can become upset or even angry. Recognizing this selfishness or feeling like too much of a burden, your adolescent may feel guilty as well. The best thing to do is to talk it out.

Talking to Your Adolescent

Understanding the needs of your adolescent can open the door to much better communication. However, if you want your discussions to be helpful, treat your adolescent like an adult. This will provide the best response. Think about your teenager's concerns about your condition. Leslie may be very frightened that her mother is never going to get better. However, her mother can help by reassuring her that her condition is fine and that she's feeling better. If your adolescent feels comfortable talking to you about your lupus, encourage it. But remember to respect the rights of those adolescents who would rather not discuss it.

Finally . . .

Your adolescent may shoulder more responsibilities because of your condition. This may cause problems, especially if your adolescent tries to deny your condition. Some adolescents will be able to deal effectively with their burdens, but some won't. They may simply be unable to handle the pressure. If your adolescent must assume any additional adult responsibilities or jobs because of your condition, consider that he or she may also be ready to enjoy some more adult privileges and pleasures. How can you require teenagers to fulfill adult responsibilities and then deny them adult privileges? If you're apprehensive about their maturity, keep in mind that if they're old enough to do adult chores, they might enjoy some adult privileges as well (within reason, of course). Adolescents will usually be more willing to help out if they know that they will be treated and trusted in a more grown-up way.

COPING WITH PARENTS

Parents usually have a very hard time dealing with any illness or condition that their child (even an adult "child") may have. Therefore, if your parents are alive, they're probably having trouble handling your lupus. This makes coping harder for you, too. Why? You don't want your parents to suffer or be upset. You'd probably feel guilty if they were suffering.

If your relationship with your parents is good, then you're among the lucky ones. But what if you normally have difficulty dealing with your parents? Having lupus doesn't help! How have your parents treated you since your diagnosis? Do they ignore or minimize your condition? Or do they smother you?

The Ignorers

Elizabeth, a 22-year-old secretary living with her parents, has had lupus for two years. Since her diagnosis, her parents have been showing less and less concern about her condition. When Elizabeth is in pain, her mother just tells her to "take her pills." When she is tired, her father tells her that "staying in bed won't accomplish anything." If looks could kill, Elizabeth's parents would be in their graves by now. Besides all of this, they don't ask questions. Even worse, they don't show any interest when she wants to tell them something about her condition.

Parents who ignore or play down your lupus often do so because they can't deal with it. They can't face the fact that their child is sick. They can't accept the possibility that it might have something to do with them. How? They may be afraid that they did something that contributed to the illness or condition. Or maybe they think you inherited the illness or condition from them.

Even if this is far from the truth, it doesn't eliminate the worry underlying such thoughts. To avoid these unpleasant feelings, they may try to deny that you have lupus. They might minimize it, hoping that it will go away.

The Smotherers

Since Alice developed lupus, her mother has visited her an average of four times per week. At first you might think that her mother's actions are very endearing. However, if you consider the following, you may change your mind: her mother lives thirty minutes away by car, has a heart condition, and needs her rest, and Alice doesn't want to see her this often. You see, Alice is 36, hasn't lived at home in seventeen years, and often disagrees with her mother's opinions (especially regarding what activities she should participate in and how much rest she should get). Alice feels that her mother is smothering her.

Parents who smother believe that if you have any kind of problem, they must take care of you. Having lupus certainly fits this requirement. It doesn't matter what your marital status is or how old you are. What matters to them is that they are your parents. They are responsible for you and must take care of you. The fact that you can take care of yourself doesn't matter. They'll call frequently to ask how you're doing. They'll want to know what they can do to help. They may come over as often as possible to make sure that you're O.K. Whether they come over or not, they'll constantly bombard you with questions about your health and activities. What can you do, short of moving out of town and taking on a new identity?

Remember what we said before? It really helps to see a situation through someone else's eyes! Don't you think this holds true here, too? Look at yourself and your condition through the eyes of your parents. How do you think they feel? What do they see? You don't have to agree with them, but understanding how they feel will help you talk to them. Looking at your condition through their eyes will also improve any discussions you may have with them, as you try to explain how you feel. It's fine to let them know that it bothers you when they do certain things. You'll feel great if your discussions are more productive.

What if Talking Doesn't Help?

If you have tried to talk to them and haven't succeeded, at least you've tried. That will help you feel a little better! At least you won't feel as if you should do more to convince them to switch to your way of thinking! What should you do then? Concentrate more on helping yourself feel better, regardless of whether they understand or not. If they're unhappy with you because you seem to be rejecting their well-meant intentions, so be it.

By the way, if you're unhappy with parents who are ignorers, you'd probably love them to smother you for awhile. And, if you don't like smothering parents, the thought of being left alone is probably very exciting. There's rarely a perfect solution. No one gets along with everyone all the time. Instead of complaining about your parents' faults, try to look at the positives in their behavior. You'll feel better about doing this, too.

How Much Should You Tell Your Parents?

You know your parents. You know how they react to things. What would you really like to share with them? Would you like to tell them how you're feeling at a particular time? You probably know how they react to good news and bad news, and how they deal with unpleasantness. How will you handle their reactions? All these factors will help you to decide how much to tell them.

Sometimes, it's easier to talk with one parent than the other. You might tell one parent what's bothering you, and let that parent tell the other. For example, your mother may be able to get through to your father better than you can. This will help everybody.

You might wish you could share unpleasant feelings with a parent because of the reassurance it would bring. It's nice to know that you don't have to face something unpleasant alone. However, what if your parents can't readily accept your problems even if they wanted to? It may be more detrimental for you to tell them things that they can't handle. So don't tell them anything impulsively. Think about and analyze the situation. Try to understand what you want to share, and what their reactions may be. It's worth the effort. By spending a little time to figure out what's best, you can help yourself feel a lot better. You'll probably improve your relationship with your parents as well.

24

Friends and Colleagues

Aside from family, the most important people you'll have to deal with are friends and colleagues. Are there any suggestions for coping with these important people? Of course!

COPING WITH YOUR FRIENDS

What reactions to your lupus have your friends had? How many of your friends really know what you're going through? They may have read about your condition, and at first, they may have thought they knew all about it. But because they weren't physically affected, they might not have been able to really understand what you were experiencing. Some wanted to learn more; some wanted to forget what little they knew.

Some friends may be very supportive—maybe *too* supportive. Other friends may not be supportive enough, something that can bother you even more. Your own mood really determines their reactions. If you don't want them around, if you don't want them close to you, or if you don't want them asking questions, and you let them know this, they will probably respect your wishes. But perhaps they won't be there when you really *do* want them around. It's important for you to strike a balance. You may simply want to explain that your feelings change and ask them to please bear with you. You can hope that they'll understand the fluctuation of your feelings.

Apprehension Keeps Them Away

Friends may not know what to say to you. What should they ask you? How should they talk to you? Their awkwardness can cause so much tension that they don't even want to be with you. They may feel so uneasy that they ask themselves, "Why bother?"

Friends may be afraid to call because they don't know how you're feeling. They don't want to run the risk of stirring up unpleasant feelings in you (or in themselves, if they don't know how to respond). On the other hand, there may be times when friends keep asking you how you're feeling and you'd really like to be left alone. Many friendships are lost or hurt because of misunderstandings. These misunderstandings usually involve uncertainty on your part or that of your friends in approaching one another.

Showing Concern

Can anything be done, or are you going to be a hermit for the rest of your life? Don't despair. There are things you can do to improve the situation. Try to set up ground rules with your friends. Tell them how you feel. If you are the kind of person who likes to be asked how you feel, let your friends know. If you'd rather not be asked, let your friends know that, too. If your feelings fluctuate (sometimes feeling talkative about your condition, but at other times reluctant to even think about it), let your friends know. Your changing feelings may be harder for your friends to deal with, so let them know that they don't have to hold back—that they can talk to you whenever they really want to. You'll let them know if and when you're having trouble.

Clear up the question marks. If you tell your friends how you feel and what your needs and desires are, fewer unknowns will exist. The uneasiness about what to do or say, which can hurt friendships, will be reduced. Your friends will become more aware of your needs, and will feel closer to you and less afraid.

Changing Plans

Don't you love having to change plans with a friend at the last minute because you're so tired that you can't even move? Probably not. So you can understand how your friends might feel if they were to have restrictions placed on their activities. This doesn't have to be so.

Good friends who understand or at least try to understand what you're going through will probably be able to accept these changes. Others may be less willing to put up with them.

Kelly hated when she and her husband made plans with friends and she had to bow out because of lupus. What made it worse was that her husband went ahead with the plans anyway! She had to stay home alone because no one else wanted to change their plans. So there was not only friction between Kelly and her friends, but increasing marital arguments as well. Since these problems are part of having lupus, you'll have to hope that discussing them with your friends will result in increased tolerance and understanding so that you can maintain some good friendships.

Asking for Help

As you learn to live with lupus, do you feel a greater need to call on your friends for help? You may need help cleaning the house, getting places, taking care of children, or purchasing groceries, among other things. Are you becoming more selfish because you ask others to do these things for you? No, but it may seem that way to you. You're asking for help more often now not out of selfishness, but because you're less able to do things independently. You'd probably like to be able to do things independently. You'd probably like to be able to do these things yourself, but it's just not possible. The reality is that there are certain things you must take care of. If they don't get done, then what will happen? So if you need help, reach out for it. That's better than pushing yourself too much and suffering the consequences. If your friends complain or show resentment, try to talk it over with them. Don't wait until a friendship is destroyed to realize that built-up problems should have been discussed earlier, when the conflict could have been resolved. If you try and nothing helps, remember this: If your friends still don't understand, what kind of friends are they, anyway?

Asking for Help Appropriately!

If you do need help, figure out who to ask and what they can do for you. If your friend Myrna loves children, it would probably be better to ask her for help with the kids. If you know that Maureen suffers from "supermarketitis," requiring daily therapeutic visits to the local food emporium, then sending her for groceries shouldn't bother her at all. If Mario has a driving phobia, don't ask him to chauffeur you around. Try to arrange for a proper fit when asking for help.

Older friendships also tend to be stronger and more resilient. Such friends will probably be more receptive if you ask for favors. Newer or more casual friends should probably not be burdened as much. Without giving a friendship a chance to become firmly planted on your hook, you may lose your prized fish—a good, solid friendship. Don't come on too strong. You might think, "But can't they see that I need help?" The answer is, "Not necessarily."

Don't feel that you must do everything yourself. There's nothing wrong with reaching out for help. But you'll feel better if you try to evaluate who would be the best person to ask to do a particular favor. (By the way, when you feel up to it, a nice way to show your appreciation is through an unsolicited gift or gesture.)

Losing Friends

What if it just doesn't work out the way you want? For example, what if people you thought were your friends don't call or visit? Some may be "turned off" by your condition. Maybe they're afraid it's contagious! Others may seem reluctant to make any plans with you, saying, "Let's wait and see how you feel." It's sad, but in some cases it just can't be avoided. It's not your decision! You may wonder if your friends reacted this way because they couldn't handle your having lupus. Were your friends uncomfortable about being with you? Were they unsure of what to say or do? Were they unable to handle the change of plans? Whatever the reason, you've probably learned a hard, unpleasant lesson. Although you may feel sad, you can't change someone else's feelings. Be reassured that most people who lose friends because of lupus do make new ones. You really don't want a friend who is uncomfortable with you.

There may be times, unfortunately, when a friend or lover cannot handle your condition and you may feel as if you've been rejected. This can be devastating! You may feel not only that you have been rejected, but that you will not be able to develop any other meaningful relationships. This is not true. You are still the same person you were before, except for the ways that lupus has affected you physically. Keep telling yourself this, so you can restore any confidence that may have been shaken by this unfortunate rejection.

Usually, however, if rejection occurs or if a relationship breaks up, it couldn't have been too strong to begin with. Many weak relationships have broken up because of medical problems. A sturdy relationship, even if it has to go through some rough times, will probably end up even stronger than before. Remember, you want a friend who likes you the way you are, lupus and all! And there are plenty of wonderful, understanding people out there. So don't give up!

COPING WITH COLLEAGUES

We've discussed some of the problems you may have working if you have lupus. If you know you're going to work, what kinds of problems might you encounter? You're going to spend several hours each day in contact with the people you work with. You'll certainly want to feel comfortable around them. Let's discuss some of the ways in which you might encounter difficulties in getting along with your colleagues.

Being There!

If you have to curtail your working hours, or if you find that you are absent from work more frequently because of lupus symptoms, you may encounter some bitterness or resentment. Nancy was a 46-year-old executive secretary who had worked in the same office for nineteen years. After being diagnosed with lupus, she found it necessary to reduce her eight-hour-a-day work schedule to four hours. This plan was endorsed by her supervisors, but was not accepted graciously by her colleagues. Many of them would have preferred working on this same kind of part-time arrangement! Your new schedule may cause bitterness and strain your working relationships. Some people just don't want to understand what's happening to you and why. They may feel that you're taking advantage of the situation. Hopefully this won't happen. For the most part, if you are comfortable with yourself, others will be too. Many colleagues will take your condition in stride and won't even think about it. This assumes, of course, that these people know about your condition. But what if you don't want to tell anyone? Unless nosy colleagues ask questions, you may decide not to bother even telling them. Obviously, there is no requirement that you do so.

Would it help to provide your colleagues with some basic information on lupus? It might, although it may not necessarily improve their attitude toward you or the disease. In addition, reading about something doesn't always lead to understanding. However, at least you'll feel better knowing that you've tried to help them understand more about lupus. If they don't, they don't. Remember: You can't change somebody else. If a colleague (or anybody else, for that matter) can't handle or understand what's going on, that's his or her problem. You can try to educate people about lupus, but don't make it your problem. If you've got an employer with an open mind, that's terrific. Don't be as concerned about other people who don't understand what you're going through. Concentrate more on doing the best you can.

Cooperative Colleague Compromises

Elaine found it impossible to complete all of her required work. She was afraid she'd lose her job. However, rather than giving up, she was able to make an arrangement with one of her colleagues who was willing to assist her in completing her tasks whenever she felt physically unable to do so alone. As a result, much of the pressure on Elaine's shoulders was removed.

Occasionally, you may find that you are less able to complete all of your work. Try to work out some kind of an arrangement with a colleague. You may feel strange (even uncomfortable) asking for help at first, but it can result in even better relationships and understanding among your colleagues. You have nothing to lose. The worst they could say is, "No! I won't help."

Employer Acceptance or Harassment?

What if you've been out of work for a while and are ready to reenter the job market? You might worry about whether you should go back to your old job, or whether anyone else would even consider hiring you. The decision to hire or not to hire you is based on a number of factors. Among them are your prior sickness or absentee record, your present state of health, and the possibility of prolonged absences in the future. The employer will certainly want to consider whether you and your medical condition will create any problems on the job. Concerns about morale, sick benefits, and liability usually top the list.

The most upsetting cases involve employers who are unwilling to hire you simply because they know about your condition. At this point, you're faced with two choices. You can either give up and look for something else, or try to educate the employer (not with your fists!). This can be done through discussions or reading materials, or you can put your employer in contact with a physician or nurse. If necessary, your physician can probably reassure your prospective employer that you're fit for the job and should be able to handle it in more or less the same way as someone without lupus.

All this groundwork is frequently worth the effort! If you do get the job, your relationship will already be a good one. Greater understanding will exist. In addition, it's nice to know that your employer has at least some insight into your condition.

Debby had been working in the same office for eight years. Because of lupus, she had been having more difficulty completing her tasks and getting to work each day. Unfortunately, her supervisor was a demanding perfectionist who apparently was not willing to bend at all for Debby. He called her in for a review and made it perfectly clear that unless her performance and attendance improved, she would be out of a job. In addition to calling her in, he frequently reminded her (in both a subtle and blunt fashion) that he was watching her. The pressure became so hard for Debby to bear that it began to affect her mental and physical health. What do you do if you feel you're being harassed?

Let's say that your employer has expressed displeasure about curtailed work time. What if an ultimatum is given, stating that if productivity does not improve, you will be discharged? (Polite, isn't he?) This is another potential problem. So what do you do? You do the best you can. If an employer doesn't understand enough about lupus to know that you must pace yourself, and shows little or no willingness to cooperate, then you're probably better off not continuing employment there. You don't want to look for trouble.

For financial reasons, should you wait until your employment is terminated? This idea has its pros and cons. If you receive unemployment benefits for losing your job, this could ease financial burdens. But if subsequent employers are reluctant to hire you because of the grounds for dismissal, is it worth it? Only you can decide, and you'll probably have to base your decision on your own unique situation. It's a very important question, since your psychological state is so important in your ability to cope with lupus. If your employment is aggravating you, then changes may have to be made.

Time to Punch Out

Whether you need to work or simply enjoy working, you'll certainly want to minimize any potential occupational problems caused by your condition. Take one day at a time. Don't worry about problems that have not and may never occur. If your lupus does cause a problem, be precise in identifying exactly what it is, so that you can employ the best strategies to resolve it.

25

Your Physician

How do you feel about your physician? (What a question!) Some people see physicians as gods. Others feel that they're rich, unconcerned, cold professionals who don't really want to help. Of course, there are other opinions. What's your feeling? This plays a role in determining how your treatment progresses. You may find that your feelings toward your physician (or physicians in general) have changed since your diagnosis. Some people with lupus don't have as much confidence in their physicians, probably because they haven't been cured yet! It may seem that physicians don't know best, and that you yourself know how you feel better than anyone else. Because of all these feelings, as well as the rising costs of medical care, physicians frequently bear the brunt of much hostility. But physicians *do* want to help. They may occasionally feel as frustrated as you do, but may not know what to suggest. It's unpleasant for anyone to admit that the answers are out of reach, especially when that person knows you are relying on him or her.

Regardless of your opinions of the medical profession, your condition makes it impossible for you to stay away from your physician. In fact, you'll have to see your physician more often than someone who is not chronically ill, so you'll want to make sure you have a good working relationship with him or her. Because you will want to understand the changes that are taking place in lupus and check with your physician when you go through flares and remissions and when your symptoms change, you'll certainly benefit from trying to develop the best possible relationship with your physician. That takes awareness, understanding, and effort on your part.

OFFICE VISITS

Since lupus can be a serious medical condition, it requires ongoing visits to your physician. These appointments aim to keep your symptoms in check, and allow your physician to carefully monitor the medication you're taking. Visits to your physician will also determine if treatment is proceeding properly.

Depending on your condition, the type of treatment you're receiving, and your physician, there may be different types of examinations during the office visit. Various tests are used to check on your health. Blood tests will probably be done frequently.

So checkups are important to keep your condition under control. Although some patients deny the possibility of any problems and try to avoid regular checkups, the intelligent person is the one who sees the doctor regularly and as "prescribed."

Make the most of your visits. Have a list of questions to ask, and jot down notes as they are answered. Doctors are usually cooperative, believing that this makes the office visit more efficient and time-effective.

BEING AFRAID OF YOUR PHYSICIAN

Are you hesitant about speaking to your physician? Perhaps you're afraid of being put in the hospital if your physician finds out how you've been feeling. You might be concerned that your physician will not like the way you're taking care of yourself. You might be afraid your doctor will consider you a complainer who's "crying wolf" and so may not take you seriously if an emergency occurs. You might be worried that your physician will increase your medication. Or you may be afraid that your physician, thinking that the symptoms you are reporting are "all in your head," won't believe what you're saying! Despite these concerns, you do want your physician to do the best for you. So try to be completely open and honest about the way you're feeling and what you're doing.

STICKING UP FOR YOUR RIGHTS

People like to believe that their physicians know what they're talking about. This doesn't mean, however, that you must blindly accept everything that's said. For the most part, physicians respect the patient who asks questions. Disagreement doesn't mean that your physician will throw you out or even back down. But if you are unsure of why something is being suggested, question your physician. If you don't like a particular medication or if it does not seem to be working for you, speak up. Don't hold back. You do have the right to question. In fact, you have the obligation to question. Uncertainty will surely make you feel tense. And relaxation is so important. . . .

GETTING SECOND OPINIONS

Because you may not absolutely agree with everything your physician says, and because no physician knows it all, you might want a second opinion. You should have a justifiable reason for seeking another opinion. But many people are worried about hurting their physician's feelings. Don't let that stop you. Think logically. Most physicians will accept your desire to get a second opinion. It will either confirm what they feel or point out the need for further discussion. If your physician objects to your getting a second opinion, you should certainly question why. This does not suggest, however, that you should make a habit of going for second opinions. Nor should you continually shop around for the "ideal" physician. No such person exists.

BEING ABLE TO REACH YOUR PHYSICIAN

Do you know what's really frustrating? How about when you call your physician for whatever reason (whether it's an emergency or not) and have to wait long hours before your call is returned? This may be one of your concerns when searching for a physician. Make sure you feel confident that your physician will promptly return your calls.

After you've lived with lupus for a while, you'll better know when you should call and when it's not necessary. Certain symptoms, such as intense pain, seizures, and a high fever, may require you to contact your physician immediately. Other symptoms, such as minor joint pains, may not have to be reported immediately. Discuss this with your physician. Find out how he or she would feel if you were to call when you were having problems. Ask about the kind of things that should be phoned in. Also ask when the best time to call would be.

YOU'RE NOT "LOCKED IN"

If you are not happy with your physician, you're not under any obligation to continue seeing him or her. Don't continue a relationship unless it's a good one. Don't continue going to a particular physician if you feel you can't ask questions, if you feel intimidated, or if you feel you can't call if there is a problem. Don't stick with your physician if you don't have confidence in what you're told, whether it's about treatment or medication. Finally, don't continue seeing your physician if you feel that he or she doesn't care about you and doesn't have your best interests at heart.

Your honesty is part of a good professional relationship. If your questions or disagreements hurt the relationship or if you are afraid of being honest, then this relationship may not be the one for you.

You may want to discuss all of this with your doctor before making any moves. You might be able to straighten things out and improve the relationship. But if you can't, remember that you're looking out for your health. You want the support of a physician who can meet most of your needs.

26

Comments From Others

As Ralph Kramden of *The Honeymooners* would say, "Some people have a *B-I-G MOUTH*!" You may agree with this when you think of some of the comments you hear from people around you. They may know you have lupus, but that doesn't mean they know how to talk to you about it or what to say. They may say things that they feel are right, witty, intelligent, or even sympathetic. But you may think otherwise! There are times when a certain comment might make you want to implant your knuckles into the speaker's teeth! Or when a comment might make you wonder if you're talking to a graduate of the Ignoramus School of Tactlessness.

But why are you reading all this? As you know by now, you cannot change other people. You cannot improve their lack of sensitivity or the way they talk. What you *can* do is learn how to cope with some of the ridiculous comments that you may hear.

ARE OTHERS BEING CRUEL?

Most people will say things out of sincere concern for you. They may be trying to make you feel better, to show their support, or to show their interest in you by asking how you feel. Does that mean you must always be receptive to their questions and respond to all of them seriously? It would be nice. The problem is that hearing the same questions over and over can begin to get on your nerves. Initially, you may try either to respond gently to comments or questions or to politely change the subject. However, these tactics do not always work. Some people avoid these annoying questions simply by not telling anyone about their condition. However, if your lupus is noticeable, certain comments may be directed toward you anyway.

For the purpose of this chapter, let's assume that we're discussing those comments that you can't avoid from the people who haven't yet learned to tune into your feelings. If you haven't heard any of these, that's great! But read on anyway. You never know when what you read might come in handy!

THREE WAYS OF RESPONDING

Many of the things that people say to you may be legitimate comments, but may bug you just the same. Others may not even deserve answers. Still others may be said without considering your feelings. But it doesn't matter why the comment is inappropriate. What really matters is that you handle these comments in a way that is comfortable for you. There are basically three ways that this can be done.

The first way is by ignoring the comments. This is not always easy, especially if the person is waiting for your response or seems genuinely insulted by your lack of response. How do you get the person to stop asking, short of buying a muzzle? Change the subject or walk away—ignore the question.

The second way is by trying to answer the questions in a rational and intelligent way, explaining your answer, how you feel, or whatever it is that you sincerely want to communicate to the other person. But now you may feel like you're banging your head against a wall. What if you just can't convince the other person of what you're trying to say? Such frustration can be painful! There's a limit to how many times you can try to explain something clearly, and not have it understood or accepted, before you explode. (And this isn't good for your physical health, either!)

What if the first two ways don't do the trick? There's got to be a better way, and there is. The third way is to respond humorously. When should you react this way? If someone says something unreasonable to you or asks you a foolish question that can't really be answered logically, you'll accomplish very little by ignoring it or trying to reasonably explain your feelings. You don't know if your answer will be accepted or if the interrogation will continue. So, in many cases, the third option may be best. The idea behind it is that the person is asking or saying something that is really unanswerable. So you're going to have a little fun with your response. You're going to say the opposite of what the person expects, a technique called "paradoxical intention." Let's see how it works.

Handling the "Big Mouth" Syndrome

What might you hear? And how should you handle it? Remember, the best response is one that will educate the "commenter." You'd like to explain your situation nicely, in a nonoffensive, sincere way. But you're only human. So how can you respond when you get fed up? Read on.

"But You Look So Good . . ."

You've awakened in the morning after a full night's sleep, but you still feel tired. You have a lot to do to get ready for your day's activities, but you don't feel like doing much of anything. Your husband walks into the room and asks you if you are ready to get up. You tell him that you're not ready yet; you'd like to rest some more because you feel really lousy. He looks at you and says, "How can you feel lousy? You look so good."

Wouldn't it be nice if you had enough energy at this point to pop him in the nose? When you don't feel well, it can be very frustrating to be told that you look good. This is one of those statements that's hard to ignore, but it's just as hard and impractical to try to explain how you feel rationally. So how can you respond to this statement humorously? You might say, "Yes, I know I look good. You can call my plastic surgeon and thank him." Or you can say, "I know I look good. Now put on your glasses and take another look." Or you can say, "Yes, I look good. Wait until you see me without my mask on." Notice that in all three cases, you are agreeing with the person first, and then you're saying something humorous. Isn't that better than saying, "How can you say I look good when I feel so awful?"

"You Look Awful!"

On the other side of the coin, it can be just as upsetting when somebody says, "Wow, you look lousy!" You may feel lousy, but you certainly don't want to be reminded of it. You surely don't want to think that the way you feel is so obvious to others. You'd like to believe that you at least look O.K. to those around you. Even if it's said sympathetically, being told that you don't look well may be insulting. So what do you say? You might respond, "Thank you, so do you!" Or, "Yes, I know. I've worked hard to look that way." Or if you're in a really cynical mood, you might say, "I know I look lousy. That comes from hearing people tell me this!" Of course, you could always say, "That makes sense, since I don't feel so hot, either!"

"Why Don't You Get Up and Do Something?"

Consider what you would do if you were in the following situation. You are sitting in a chair relaxing because you really feel exhausted and want some peace and quiet. Somebody comes over to you and asks what's wrong. You try to explain that you're feeling very tired and are trying to gather some energy. Obviously trying to show his or her concern for you and to be helpful, the person says, "You're spending too much time thinking about yourself. Just get up and do something. Soon you won't even remember that you're not feeling well!" How do you react to this view of your condition? Do you jump out of your chair? Of course not. If you had the energy to get out of your chair, you wouldn't have been slumped there in the first place. Should you sit there and try to explain that you are feeling lousy? No, because the person probably won't believe you. So how do you respond humorously? You might say, "I would like to get up, but somebody put fast-drying glue on the chair, and I'm stuck forever!" Or you might respond, "I'm trying to set a Guinness world record for the most time I can spend in this chair." Or you might say, "Do you know how much energy it takes to remain in this chair, when what I really want to do is to get up and knock your block off?" Obviously, the type of response you use depends on how angry or irritated you feel. Remember: For this approach to work best, you want to respond in a lighthearted way. This will show the person making the comment that you're fine, but you just don't appreciate what he or she is saying.

"Too Many Doctors Will Spoil Your Mind"

Let's say a friend finds out that you have yet another doctor's appointment. You may hear, "You're just going to too many doctors. Why don't you stop going all over the place and just do what you have to do?'' How do you respond to this? You might respond by saying, ''Yes, and I'll keep going to different doctors until I exhaust my bank account.'' Or you might say, ''I like to go to a lot of doctors. The smell of the antiseptic waiting room excites me!'' Or, ''Do you realize how many of their children I'm putting through college this way?''

''What Did You Do to Yourself?''

Some people are convinced that whenever something goes wrong, it is a result of personal neglect. Let's say you're having a lot of pain in your legs. As a result, when you try to walk, you're moving much more gingerly and uncomfortably than usual. You meet a friend in the street who says, ''What did you do to your leg?'' This kind of question usually does show genuine concern. Under some circumstances, you might simply want to explain that your pain is keeping you from walking properly. But if this is the twenty-fourth time you've heard the same question, it may be harder to respond calmly. What could you say that would not be cruel, but which would still allow you to feel better about the way you handled the situation? How about, ''This isn't my leg. This is the wooden leg I got from the lumberyard!'' Or, ''Normally I walk better than this, but I just finished a marathon dance contest.'' Or you could say, ''I'm injured from kicking people who keep asking me what I did to myself!'' This does not suggest that you be unfeeling in your answers. However, if you need to let the ''commenter'' know that you don't appreciate these questions, that'll do it!

''How Can You Stand So Much Pain?''

In response to this profoundly sympathetic expression of curiosity, you might want to ask, ''What pain? The pain from my joints or the pain I get from these dumb questions!'' Or you might want to point out other feelings, such as, ''I've grown rather accustomed to not being able to move!'' Or you might simply say, ''I don't stand it. I usually have to lie down!'' People will get the message. You may not like the pain of lupus, but at least you're learning to cope with it.

''What's Lupus?''

How do you respond if somebody says, ''I never heard of lupus''? You might say, ''Let's forget you even brought it up. Then you can keep your streak going!'' Or you could say, "I never heard of it either. How's the weather?'' Don't forget: You really don't want to hurt the person's feelings by being sarcastic. However, coping with comments from others can be one of the hardest things about living with lupus. There are times when being gentle and tactful with others is less important than helping yourself to handle comments without becoming aggravated.

If the person asks why you sound sarcastic, you can explain that you're not trying to be that way. But the comment you just heard was so ridiculous that you figured the person was trying to be funny. So you decided to have some fun, too! But if the person really wants to know how you feel . . .

You won't always have to use this technique, but you may want to be prepared to use it anyway. You'll always come across someone who will say or ask something ridiculous. However, as you learn to feel better about your responses to comments, you'll find that you can handle them more calmly. You won't have to use sarcastic-type comments, and you'll have more fun with humorous, enjoyable ones. You'll keep people on your "friend" list rather than on your "you know what" list.

What if you're thinking, "I could *never* say those things. It's just not my style.'' Well, you don't always have to. But you can at least *think* these comments. Even that will help you to feel better!

OTHER LOVABLE COMMENTS

What are some of the other comments that you may hear? How many of these have come your way? "Is lupus contagious?'' "Is lupus a form of cancer?'' "Why don't you quit your job?'' "You should exercise more!'' "Are you sure you can walk up those stairs?'' "Go sit in the sun for a while!'' "Rest. Don't do anything.'' "What did the doctor say?'' "Why does your face look that way?'' "What is the prognosis?'' "Wow, have you changed!'' "You must miss the way things used to be.'' "What's the matter with you?'' "Can I help you?'' "I certainly don't envy you.'' "If you would eat right, you'd feel better!'' "Why don't you try my doctor?'' "Your having lupus is the worst thing I ever heard!''

IS THAT ALL?

Volumes would be needed to include all of the comments that you might hear from well-meaning friends or relatives. By reading these examples, you can at least get an idea of how to respond in a humorous way. Look over this list. Can you come up with some goodies? You don't want to be cynical or cruel. Rather, you want to show the speaker that you're feeling well enough to respond lightheartedly.

A FINAL COMMENT

One of the most common and yet most irritating comments that you may hear has been saved for last. Imagine that somebody who is supposedly sympathetic and trying to help you feel better turns to you with eyes full of compassion and concern, and says, "I heard about someone who died from lupus!" As you turn to walk away, you respond, "I heard about someone who was killed after telling someone with lupus what you just told me!" You walk away with your head held high and a smile on your face, leaving the astonished well-wisher behind you.

27

Sex and Lupus

This chapter is *not* rated R, for Restricted. Rather, it is rated E, for Essential. Why? If you are sexually active, living with lupus can certainly have an impact on your sex life.

Has lupus decreased your sexual appetite or ability? This can have an important bearing on the closeness of the relationship with your partner. What kind of sexual relationship did you have before you were diagnosed? (I'm not being nosy. You don't have to write and tell me!) Was it a solid one, or was it on shaky ground? If you had a good sexual relationship, you'll have an easier time getting over any obstacles that lupus may have thrown into your sex life. If your sexual relationship wasn't good, it is unlikely that having lupus will make it better. You may need some professional help to keep things from breaking down altogether. But don't lose hope. If you unite with your partner to work things out together—reassuring each other, relearning how to please each other, and showing a desire for each other—progress can certainly be made.

WHERE'S THE PROBLEM?

Let's talk about what the problems might be. There can be both physiological and psychological reasons for changes in your sexual appetite. Physiological problems are better suited to specific treatments. Psychological problems are harder to deal with (ah, there's the rub). Let's explore some of the different possibilities.

The Body Beautiful? (Physical Problems)

Can physical problems alter your interest in sex? You bet your hormones they can!

There is no question that lupus can have an effect on your sex life. What can cause some of the difficulties? Several symptoms of lupus may get in the way. If you have pain in your joints, are you going to want to move around? Probably not. Sexual activity, offset by pain, is not too pleasant, causing the "ooh, ouch syndrome."

Because painful movement or restriction of joints can make sex difficult, it's important to explore possible ways of changing this. Try procedures that can help relax your muscles or reduce pain, such as moist heat, warm baths, or compresses. Limbering-up exercises may pave the way to more pleasurable sexual encounters. (This gives new meaning to the word "warm-up," doesn't it?)

You may want to try different positions. Some of them may put less of a strain on problem joints. If sexual activity is painful, you may be better off taking a more passive role in your encounters. Assume a less active position. On occasion, the use of simple devices such as pillows or knee pads can make sex a lot less painful.

Is there any particular time of day when you experience less pain? For some people, it may be too uncomfortable to have sex late at night. Others may be too stiff in the morning or the early part of the day. Working these problems out takes the cooperation of both partners. Kids, work, and other responsibilities may interfere, of course, but it's better to have sex at planned times than not at all. Frequently, sexual problems can be helped by using your imagination and experimenting with different varieties (in position, timing, and technique).

Fatigue can be a factor in the frequency with which you engage in sex. If you're tired, you're going to be less interested in sexual activity. This can be a real headache! (Sorry about that!) But if you're uncomfortable or fatigued, hanky-panky will just have to be put on hold. Is this a poor choice of words? Actually, it may be an excellent idea. After all, just holding each other can be a wonderful experience, too!

Raynaud's phenomenon may reduce sexual interest as well. With Raynaud's, circulation of blood is restricted in the extremities. During sexual excitement, more blood concentrates in the genital area, further reducing the amount of blood that is available to the fingers and toes, and creating a lot of pain in these extremities. You certainly don't want to hurt during sex. What fun is that? The use of medication, even aspirin, can help both joint pain and Raynaud's phenomenon. A warm bath can be very soothing, and a nice waker-upper to prepare you for a pleasurable sexual encounter. Raise the temperature in the bedroom. This can improve blood circulation in the hands and toes, adding to your comfort.

What about drugs? Sexual problems may be caused by such medication as painkillers, sedatives, and tranquilizers, or by other types of "drugs" like alcohol. It's true that small amounts of these may make you feel more relaxed (increasing the possibility of sex), but too much can work against you. The use of alcohol is notorious in reducing sexual abilities because of its effect on the body.

Some drugs can have a direct effect on sexual desire. For example, certain medication (such as tranquilizers, which reduce your anxiety) can suppress sexual desire or your ability to achieve orgasm. Antihypertensive medication may also have an effect on sexual performance.

How do mouth or vaginal ulcers or sores interfere with sex? Although painful, these ulcers don't forbid all kinds of sexual activity. Certain types of nonulcer-inhibited physical contact can be enjoyed as long as both partners are willing. A warm, understanding relationship certainly makes this possible. But ulcers can be treated. Treatments include steroid applications, such as special mouthwashes with added antibiotics, for mouth ulcers, and steroid suppositories for treating vaginal ulcers.

Some women may experience dryness. The dryness may be in your mouth, eyes, or vagina (Sjögren's syndrome). This can be a problem. Vaginal dryness can make intercourse so painful that you'll want to avoid it. (It may also cause bleeding.) But don't think of vaginal dryness as a lack of excitation. Dryness is not an unusual complication of lupus. If dryness causes painful intercourse, what can you do? Keep in mind that a longer period of foreplay can increase vaginal lubrication. Otherwise, consider using water-soluble lubricants such as KY jelly. This can ease the dryness that might otherwise interfere with or prevent sexual activity.

Going Out of Your Head? (Psychological Problems)

Your body isn't the only thing that may affect your sexual interest. Your mind also comes into the picture.

What's the most important sex organ? Think hard now. The correct response is your brain! (Did I catch you?) If a sexual problem exists that is not physiological, then it doesn't exist in your body, but in your mind.

Many people with lupus experience a decreased interest in sex. This doesn't necessarily mean there's something wrong with you. As a matter of fact, decreased sexual interest is common in many chronic illnesses.

Self (and Body) Image

Living with lupus may affect your self-esteem. Do you like yourself less because of your condition? If you feel this way, you may be more fearful of rejection by your partner. As a result, you may reduce sexual activity simply to minimize the chances of rejection.

Because self-esteem is a necessary factor in enjoying sexual intimacy, you'll want to improve your ability to like yourself. Feeling good about yourself and your body are very important if you want to enjoy your sexual relationships. It will also make your partner feel more comfortable. On the other hand, if you don't feel good about yourself, this will also affect your partner. This can certainly interfere with closeness!

Your perception of your body can greatly affect your self-esteem. Loss of satisfaction with your own body can decrease your self-esteem. You may feel reluctant to share your body with your spouse or partner. Do you see your body in a distorted way? Alice, a 47-year-old woman married for twenty years, was upset about her bloated appearance from long-term prednisone use. She feared that her husband would not want to touch her because of the way she looked. Do you fear that your partner may be less interested in sex because of the way you look? Actually, your partner may not feel this way. But you may try to avoid sex anyway, rather than risk rejection.

Self-consciousness can be a big problem. Some people with lupus feel less feminine or masculine because of changes in the way they move or look. How has your condition affected your perception of your sexuality? If having lupus makes you feel less sexually attractive (and interestingly, this is not uncommon), then you've targeted an important area to work on. See what things you can change (consider getting advice about clothes, make-up, and other "appearance enhancers"). Try to remember that nobody's perfect. Everybody has flaws. It makes sense to work on enhancing your looks in whatever ways are appropriate. If you are overweight, wear fashions that will trim down your appearance. If you have a big nose, apply make-up so as to give the illusion of a slimmer one. Whatever the problem, there is usually a way to correct it. But improving your mental attitude is just as important. For those problems that can't be modified, use some of the thought-changing procedures described earlier in Chapters 6, 8, and 9. They may be the key to your future happiness!

Emotional Interference

Emotions can get in the way, too! Sexual activity may be restricted because of depression. You may be so withdrawn that you simply have no interest in it. Your anxiety concerning sex itself, the intimacy of your relationship, or your sexual performance can also hold you back. You may be afraid that you just can't "make it."

Any of these things can happen to anyone—not just to people with lupus. Fortunately, they can also be changed with proper awareness, interaction, improved communication, and therapy (if necessary).

Fear may also be a factor in your ability to enjoy sex. If you are afraid of becoming pregnant, you may have a hard time enjoying spontaneous sex. Having lupus can make this fear even greater. Why? You may be concerned that your child will develop lupus! Remember, lupus is not considered to be a hereditary disease. Although small percentages of newborns may have lupus cells in their systems, these lupus cells tend to pass out of their systems within six to eight weeks following delivery. So fear of giving birth to a child with lupus need not be a reason to curtail sexual activity.

Let's say you just don't want to get pregnant. This creates a new problem: which contraceptive devices to use. Birth control pills should not be used because they can worsen a lupus condition or cause flares. Intrauterine devices (IUDs) should not be used because they also increase your chances of infection. You always want to minimize this. Many women with lupus prefer to use spermicidal jellies, foams, or creams. These preparations may not be as effective as birth control pills, but when used in combination with male contraceptive devices (such as condoms), they can minimize your chances of an unwanted pregnancy.

Pain or, more importantly, your fear of pain may decrease your interest in sex. For example, if you've had vaginal ulcers, they usually go away with proper treatment. But what if you have a long memory of the pain you suffered from ulcers, and you worry that the friction of intercourse may bring about a recurrence of ulcers? If so, the psychological effects of the ulcer may last longer than the physiological effects.

Sexual problems can be frustrating, especially if you don't have a partner. It may be uncomfortable for you to even think about finding someone new, knowing the problems you're having with lupus. Take things one step at a time. Be more social, look to make new friends, and try not to worry about the more intimate activities that might occur in the future.

TALK IT OVER

A very important part of sexual relationships is communication. If you and your partner can share thoughts and feelings, you'll be in much better shape to work out any sexual problems that may occur as a result of your condition. If communication problems exist, however, difficulties may be very hard to resolve.

It is important to discuss sexual problems with your partner. Ruth, a 38-year-old housewife, had lupus. Her husband Bill felt incapable as her lover because he was unable to get Ruth excited, and because he caused her pain whenever he attempted to make love to her. But Bill may be reassured to know that these problems could result from lupus rather than his inadequacy as a lover. If that's the case, then both Ruth and Bill should explore different methods of igniting sexual fires. Otherwise, unpleasant feelings may develop between them. You can work through such feelings, however. Acknowledge the problem and discuss it with your partner. It can be very helpful to discuss any problems with your physician or other health professional as well. In many cases, the major problem is that you keep these feelings inside, avoid discussing them, and cause your sex life to dwindle down to nothing.

Try to maintain open lines of communication with your partner. Discuss any sexual problems openly. You may even want to discuss them with your physician or another professional to determine whether they are physiological or psychological. You'll then be better able to work on them.

All that has been said, of course, assumes that your interest in sex is affected by your condition, and that your partner is suffering. But what if the opposite is true? What if you still have normal sexual desires, but your partner is the one who's afraid? Maybe your partner fears hurting you or creating additional problems. Or maybe you're regarded as a fragile flower that is easily broken, and your partner is reluctant to be sexually spontaneous. This must be carefully discussed. If one-on-one attempts at working things out don't help, don't hesitate to get some professional assistance. It's well worth it.

AND NOW THE CLIMAX

Because sex is such an intimate and important part of a marriage (or any serious relationship), the whole relationship can be affected when either or both partners feel there is trouble. Try to discuss this. If necessary, include your physician in a discussion to clarify issues that may not be as readily accepted. You can still have a warm relationship even if your sex life is less active, but not if there are bitter feelings and misgivings at the same time. Understanding each other's feelings is a very important part of coping with lupus.

Remember: Having lupus doesn't mean that sexual activity must be reduced, curtailed, or totally eliminated! As a matter of fact, it can still be as pleasurable and as important as the partners want it to be. (By the way, as long as we're talking about the climax, are you aware that orgasm triggers a release of naturally produced painkillers? What a pleasurable way to reduce pain!)

28

Pregnancy

To have a baby, or not to have a baby: that is the conception. Whether it is nobler (or safer) to have children may be a big question mark. Why? You may be concerned that if lupus is genetically transmitted, your children may have a greater chance of developing it. You may be afraid that lupus may cause a difficult or unsafe pregnancy. Let's consider some of the important issues regarding pregnancy.

DOES PREGNANCY AFFECT YOUR LUPUS?

Pregnancy can place additional stress on you, although it is impossible to predict what will happen during anyone's pregnancy. It's possible that you'll feel better than usual during your pregnancy. Or you may experience more marked symptoms and be in a flare for almost the whole time. As a matter of fact, some people first learn that they have lupus during or after their pregnancy. Why? Because symptoms develop that prompt them to go to the doctor, and voilà, they discover that they have lupus! In more than half of women with lupus, however, pregnancy has no bearing at all on the way lupus affects them. For the most part, be reassured that even if pregnancy does affect your lupus (either during or after the pregnancy), these problems are rarely so serious as to be life threatening.

Yvonne, a 25-year-old mother of one, was one of the unfortunate ones. She had been diagnosed with lupus two years prior to her current pregnancy. She was feeling pretty good, though, so she decided to add to her family. However, within two weeks of conception, she went into a flare that made her want to crawl into a washing machine and spin dry! She then considered aborting the pregnancy, hoping this would end the flare. However, in most cases, physicians feel that having an abortion will not help a flare. If anything, it may even make it worse. Physicians prefer that you take steroids to try to control the flare.

DOES LUPUS AFFECT YOUR PREGNANCY?

Unfortunately, your pregnancy may not be without problems if you have lupus. Individuals with lupus have a statistically greater chance of premature births and neonatal complications. There is a greater chance of miscarriage, and there might be a somewhat higher number of stillbirths. Despite these facts, it has not yet been clearly determined whether these problems are directly related to having lupus. The best advice? Discuss all these issues with your doctor(s).

Besides these problems, other things that can disrupt any normal pregnancy can still occur. Such pleasures as morning sickness, nausea, and fatigue are still possible. Thrilling, right?

CONCEIVING

Will you have more difficulty conceiving because of lupus? Probably not, although some women have problems conceiving regardless of their medical condition. In some cases menstruation may cease, or periods may become irregular when they used to be regular. However, physicians have indicated that even if menstruation ceases, ovulation can still take place, and conception can still occur. So if you are not menstruating, that does not mean you cannot become pregnant. Therefore, you should take normal precautions even if you're not menstruating.

When you and your spouse decide to try to have children, check with your physician to make sure there are no other reasons to hold off. For example, it's probably not a good idea to attempt to conceive while you're in the middle of a lupus flare. This doesn't mean that you can't try, however, or that something will go wrong if you conceive while in a flare. But you'll probably want your condition to stabilize so you'll be in the best possible shape for your pregnancy if it does happen. Should you try to conceive if you have elevated blood pressure or kidney involvement? Again, it's probably not the best idea, especially if your kidney trouble is severe. But speak to your doctor. Each case should be discussed individually. (In addition, you might not want to consider expanding your family if you're having difficulty fulfilling all of your current responsibilities.)

Are you concerned that there may be a possible genetic factor involved in lupus? You may be concerned about passing lupus on to your children. Although there are families in which several members have lupus, it has never been clearly proven that lupus is transmitted genetically. Most cases of lupus do not seem to be inherited. At best (or at worst?), there are some who believe that a person may be born with a susceptibility to lupus, but that it still takes something to trigger the disease—that something must happen for it to develop. So relax.

IF YOU DO CONCEIVE

If you do become pregnant, it is essential to remain in close contact with your doctor. This is especially important because you have lupus. This way, if any problems do develop, you'll be able to "nip them in the bud."

Although you may have had an obstetrician before you were diagnosed with lupus, be sure that he or she will take care of you now, considering your medical condition. Some may prefer not to treat individuals with lupus and will suggest switching to a different obstetrician. Is this unfair? You may not be happy about it, but you certainly want to know if a physician feels uncomfortable.

MEDICATION AND PREGNANCY

If you can, it's usually a good idea to avoid most medication during pregnancy. But this is not always possible. Aspirin, for example, has been used by many women during their pregnancies, without any damage to the fetus. Other medication, such as prednisone, has been used during pregnancy.

There are certain medications that shouldn't even be considered during pregnancy, such as the immunosuppressive drugs. If you're on any of these, don't even attempt to conceive yet. Wait for your doctor's go-ahead after discontinuing their use.

In all cases, don't take decisions regarding medication and pregnancy lightly. And, even more importantly, don't take decisions into your own hands. That's what you have a doctor for, right?

What if you discover that you're pregnant while you're on medication? Your doctor may want you to stop the medication as soon as possible. It's O.K. to stop some medicines abruptly. But remember that it is possible that you may have a flare-up after discontinuing their use.

Whether or not you should continue medication, stop it, or even consider pregnancy is a matter that you'll want to discuss with your family and your doctors (not just your rheumatologist, but your obstetrician and maybe even someone involved in high-risk pregnancies).

THE STORK ARRIVES

To try to avoid flares resulting from delivery, steroids are usually increased just prior to delivery. You should also try hard to avoid any stressful circumstances (other than contractions!) because of your increased vulnerability at this time.

If you do go into a flare, it may occur in the short period of time (anywhere from two weeks to two months) following delivery (the postpartum period). Increased lupus problems often relate to kidney problems or emotional distress, although flares can occur for any reason. However, close cooperation with your physician can probably reduce the likelihood of such a postpartum flare or at least of such a flare becoming serious.

WHAT ABOUT THE BABY?

In general, the babies of mothers with lupus do not show any more evidence of lupus at birth than the babies delivered by women who don't have lupus. Newborns of mothers who have lupus, however, may show a higher incidence of congenital heart block. This medical problem is usually associated with the presence of one of the antinuclear antibodies in the mother, called anti-Ro. Therefore, experts feel it would be reasonable to check all newborns of mothers with lupus for this problem so that appropriate treatment can be begun, if necessary.

If your baby was tested for the presence of LE cells or given an ANA test when born, these tests might come back positive. But the results are most likely positive because the mother's blood has been circulating within the baby. The tests usually no longer show a positive result after the baby is a few months old.

One other recommendation: If you have more than just a mild case of lupus, or if you have been on moderate dosages of steroids for prolonged periods of time, you probably shouldn't breastfeed your baby. There's no clear proof as to whether it will cause any problems, but it does take time and energy, which may fatigue you, and you don't want to pass your medication (steroids or others) to your baby in the milk.

ARE YOU PACIFIED?

As you can see, there are plenty of questions to ask yourself before deciding whether you should become pregnant. You may have questions about your medication or feel selfish or guilty about your decision to have or not to have a baby. You may worry that you really won't be able to care for the baby if your lupus is so bad that you can't hold, diaper, or feed him or her.

The best thing to do is to bring all of the issues that concern you out into the open and discuss them husband and wife, doctor and family, and obstetrician and rheumatologist. Everyone must get involved in the discussion. We're not dealing with simple questions such as, "Should I take two aspirin today or one?" We're talking about major considerations that have significant psychological overtones, too. Remember that in most cases, pregnancy should not be a problem at all, especially if you have only a mild case of lupus. What are the keys to a successful pregnancy? Awareness, supervision, and careful planning. Take all these factors into consideration, and then— good luck!

PART V
Living With Someone With Lupus

29

Living With Someone
With Lupus—
An Introduction

Illness can create changes in relationships. No kidding! If you live with someone who has lupus, you may have a number of concerns. You may now see that person differently. Maybe you are reminded of your own vulnerability. Maybe you had been dependent on that person, but now you have to shoulder more of the burden. What does all this mean? Although you share the concerns of the individual who has lupus, you also worry about yourself. If you have difficulty dealing with your loved one because of lupus, you're not alone. Illness in a loved one often creates a lot of ambivalent feelings in yourself. Concerns about the future, your loved one's health, and money may be troublesome to you. This is not unusual.

What if you feel anger toward this person, not because of anything that was done, but because of the fact that lupus has created changes? This is normal, but may still produce guilt. Why? Because this anger is directed toward somebody who, at the present time, is vulnerable and unable to defend himself or herself. (By the way, throughout this book I have purposely avoided calling the person with lupus a "patient," simply because I believe in emphasizing the person rather than the condition. However, for the sake of convenience and because repeating "your loved one" can become tedious, in this chapter I will refer to the person with lupus as the patient.)

WHAT CAN YOU DO?

If you are close to someone with lupus, you have an important job on your hands. This job is made up of many components, the most important of which is the need to be understanding and supportive. This is very important, whether you live in the same house as the patient or are simply a relative or friend. Remember: People with lupus do not have it easy, but they'll have a much harder time if they feel alone and isolated.

Learn About Lupus

A great way for you to help is by learning as much as you possibly can about lupus and its treatment. Do you enjoy worrying? You may have unnecessary worries if you don't know things about lupus treatment that the patient does. By understanding the patient's program, you can better provide support and understanding.

Know When to Let Go

Don't stay on top of the patient. Sure, you'll want to help. But give the patient enough space to regain some control over his or her own life.

How about doctor's visits? If the patient agrees, you may want to go along for the ride. There may be times when the doctor might want to discuss something with you. It might be a good idea for four ears rather than two ears to listen when the doctor is explaining lupus, medication, or other aspects of living with the disease. However, if the patient wants to go alone and feels strongly about it, don't force the issue.

Encourage, Don't Pester

Encourage adherence to proper management routines and medication needs. But don't badger. If your loved one is not taking proper care of himself or herself, there is a limit as to how much you can do to change things. Screaming usually doesn't help (and it can hurt your vocal cords!). Should you tell the physician if the patient is not taking care of himself or herself? That's a hard question to answer. You don't want to overstep your bounds and be resented. At the same time, you don't want to sit back and let the patient create unnecessary problems. This is especially true if the patient doesn't seem to care. What do you do if the patient just "gives up"? Play each situation by ear. Before deciding whether to say anything to the physician, you should discuss the situation with the patient. Voice your concerns; mention that you're afraid of a problem becoming worse. Listen to the responses before deciding whether to carry it any further.

Try to become aware of what can trigger a flare, so you can help the patient avoid these situations. Let's say, for example, that you have decided to go to the beach. If you know that the patient cannot take sun exposure, don't rub it in. Either don't go or go without calling so much attention to yourself that the patient feels uncomfortable. By all means, don't say things like, "Oh, why don't you go, you'll be O.K.!"

Sympathize, Don't Pity

Because of the difficulties that accompany lupus and its treatment, you may sympathize with the patient. You may feel sad about what he or she has to go through. This may help you to provide beneficial support. But don't pity the patient. This can be destructive.

There will be times when the patient is so fatigued that little or nothing can be done. At such times, it is not appropriate for you to insist that the person "get up and do something." That won't make him or her feel better! Try to help out. Try to reduce the patient's pressures at that time. See if you can take over any of his or her obligations or responsibilities to ease the patient's load.

At the same time, don't allow the patient to baby himself or herself. In general, if the patient can do something (even if it takes time), let the person do it. If you feel that the patient is "copping out" or malingering, you should discuss this individual's behavior with him or her. Try to make life as normal as possible for the patient.

Don't Be Extreme

Frequently, friends or relatives go from one extreme to the other. What does this mean? Of course, you'll want to help out when the patient gets tired. But when the person is no longer tired, will you allow him or her to do what is desired? When feeling better and able to do things, the last thing the patient wants is to be told to get into bed and rest. Have faith in your special someone. If the patient really doesn't feel well, he or she will rest. Otherwise, let up!

THE LONG VERSUS THE SHORT OF IT

If a patient has an acute problem, such as a heart attack, a specific treatable illness, or a broken bone, it's a lot easier for friends and relatives to rally around and to provide support and understanding, taking over the responsibilities for the patient while rehabilitation and healing are taking place. More problems occur with a chronic condition. Sure, there is a period of time when lifestyle has to be reorganized and responsibilities reassigned. But once these changes start to take place, feelings and rough spots stabilize. Life goes on.

But adjusting to a chronic condition such as lupus is harder than dealing with many other illnesses because lupus is cyclical. There are times when the patient may not be able to do much of anything and you will have to help out. At other times, during remission for example, your loved one can do a lot more, so the family now has to readjust to different roles—roles that may be similar to the ones everyone had before lupus. These cyclical changes can create major problems. Because there is no definite time when the patient is going to get better, you may have a difficult time dealing with changes in his or her condition. "This roller coaster is going to go on forever," you may think disgustedly.

HOW TO RESPOND

Can you always be sure of what the best response is for the patient? You may feel that at certain times, the best way to respond is with sympathy and understanding. At other times, the best thing may be to just ignore what's going on and walk away. There may be times when you want to joke about lupus. But there's no way for you to know for sure. You can't predict the patient's needs. How can you help? Lay ground rules. Hopefully, the patient will initiate this. If not, maybe you can start the discussion. Mention your concerns. Talk about your interest in being as helpful as you possibly can, and ask what you can do to help. Things will move more smoothly if you have a good idea of what to do and when to do it. Even if there are no clear-cut, definite answers, at least there will be some constructive communication. You'll be better able to handle future problems.

KEEP TALKING

It is very important to have open lines of communication between you and the patient. This is really the only way you can become aware of his or her physical and emotional conditions. If you do listen to the patient, you can truly help. This doesn't mean that the conversations will always be pleasant. Talking about problems, depression, fears, and joint pain isn't very enjoyable, especially if you don't have any answers. But with good communication, any difficulties will be overshadowed by the feeling of closeness resulting from shared feelings and concerns.

30

The Child With Lupus

It is not common for a child to have lupus. But if it happens, it is very likely that the doctor doing the diagnosing will immediately have two or three new patients: the child and the child's mother and/or father. This may be only the tip of the iceberg. When a child is diagnosed with a serious illness, it can have a devastating effect on the child's family. It's important for family members to work through any emotional difficulties they may experience as a result of the child's diagnosis. Communication will keep the family intact and will help the child cope with his or her condition. Who else is involved? Friends, teachers, and other relatives may all be affected by the child's condition.

THE CHILD'S PARENTS

The parents of a child diagnosed with lupus will probably experience a whole range of emotional reactions. Feelings of guilt and intense anguish are not uncommon. They may feel that their child inherited the illness from them, although this is unlikely. They may worry that they did not use the right physicians, or that they didn't take proper care of the child. "Is there something we could have done to prevent this?" parents may exclaim. All of these doubts are not uncommon. Parents are emotional after the initial diagnosis, but their worries can be destructive unless they are worked through. Parents should attempt not to communicate their fears to the child. Nor should parents make the child feel ashamed.

Watching your child experience the symptoms of lupus can be horrible. It's also hard for you to make sure that your child takes all the necessary medication and gets enough rest.

HOW TO TREAT THE CHILD

You don't want to make things harder for the child with lupus. So don't behave any differently from the way you did before the diagnosis. Don't think you have to be stricter and discipline your child more, or be more lax and indulge your child more. If you would really rather help the child adjust, then treat the child as a child, not as an unfortunate youngster with lupus. Avoid changing the way you raise your child if you want the child to be well-adjusted.

Try not to let the child see your pain or unhappiness. Imagine how the child will feel seeing unhappiness in loved ones. You can be sure the child will feel guilty. This will only make things worse.

The brothers and sisters of the child with lupus who still live at home will definitely be affected. The degree to which siblings are affected varies, however, depending on how much extra attention the child with lupus receives and how brothers and sisters react to this extra attention. Do the other siblings feel as if they're losing time with you or other relatives? They may feel that their needs are second to those of the sick sibling. This can cause tension between the child with lupus and your other children. Brothers and sisters may become resentful of the extra attention given to the ill sibling. They may not believe that lupus is such a big deal, but think that it is being blown out of proportion for extra attention. On the other hand, the child with lupus may not even want all this attention, and may feel guilty about getting it at the expense of brothers and sisters.

A CHILD WITH LUPUS, NOT A LUPUS CHILD!

Emphasize the child rather than the illness. It is better to still think of or talk about your child as a child—a child who happens to have lupus. In addition, try to maintain a calm, emotionally stable home. This is crucial to keeping the family together. It is harder to change the behavior of more distant family members. How can you communicate to friends and relatives that you don't want them to bring gifts or to shower extra attention on your child? You want your child to be treated like any other child, despite the condition.

As we've said before, parents (as well as others who are close to the child) should learn as much as possible about lupus. The more knowledge you have, the more understanding you can be. You can then be more supportive of your child.

THE CHILD CAN HELP HIMSELF OR HERSELF, TOO

Managing your child's lupus should be done matter-of-factly. Make it a regular part of life. It's usually not a good idea to reward your child just for routinely following the lupus treatment. You want the child to learn proper self-care habits—not to expect a reward. But the child will be duly rewarded for proper self-care; his or her condition will improve. Once a child's flare is controlled, remissions can usually be maintained more easily than they can in adults.

Family routines should continue as before. You all have to learn to live with any restrictions that lupus may impose. Hopefully, everyone in the family, especially the ill child, will feel at ease with your child's primary physician. You want to be confident that the physician can address any of your questions or concerns. Children, especially very young ones, will be less able than adults to understand the facts about lupus. Your child may ask, "Why do I have to go through all this?" "Why do I have to take all these pills?" "Why do I always hurt so much?" "Why can't we go to the beach anymore or go out in the sun? Why do I always have to put that stuff on when we're going outside?" "Why can't I do a lot of what I used to? Why do I have to rest so much?" Other questions may also occur. You want your child to be able to ask questions, even if you can't provide all of the answers.

HOW DO CHILDREN COPE?

An important factor in determining how well a child will adjust to lupus and its treatment is how well the child handled stress before the onset of the condition. (Does this sound familiar? Of course. This also helps determine how adults will adjust to lupus!) But having lupus is very difficult for a child, especially if physical restrictions interfere with normal activities. You'll want to do everything you can to help the child deal with this. Other problems that may occur for adults, such as feelings of isolation, pain, unhappiness with their bodies, and the side effects of medication, can also plague children. So how do children react to their condition? Some withdraw, sleeping as much as they can, staying away from friends (and even family), and keeping their bodies covered at all times. Others are very open about their condition. They almost flaunt it, trying to get extra attention. But most children with lupus fall somewhere between these two extremes.

Some children can be encouraged to learn other enjoyable activities. Swimming is a great sport, and may be good for your child's body. If your doctor approves of this activity, why not encourage it? Other nonphysical activities, such as chess or arts and crafts, can be good outlets. And, of course, doing well academically and developing good reading skills can be a great boost psychologically.

Children Deny, Too!

Children may try to deny some aspects of having lupus. They may fight fatigue, trying to do everything they used to. Or they may "forget" to take their pills. So children may deny that they have a problem. But ignoring their illness won't help it go away.

You want your child to do what's best. But there are times when children may be able to do more than you think they can. In many cases, children are less sensitive to pain and other negative aspects of the illness than adults. You may often be more concerned than your child about the lupus. Try not to be overprotective. However, you should still guide your child in the right direction. Even when your child pushes too hard, try to let the child learn for himself or herself what can and cannot be done. In order to mature while having lupus, your child must be aware of the limitations that exist.

Lashing Out

Rebellion against authority is a normal part of a child's development. When it happens, be sure that you are prepared to deal with it. At the same time, be assured that a child with lupus will probably not seriously hurt himself or herself with tantrum behavior. So deal with rebellion the same way you would if your child didn't have lupus. Ignore it, wait until the child has calmed down, and then talk to your child. However, if your child throws things around or hurts himself or herself, do try to minimize the physical effects of these outbursts. Try to keep the home environment emotionally calm, stable, supportive, and loving.

31

The Adolescent
With Lupus

Ah, the joys of adolescence! Adolescence can be one of the most difficult periods in one's life. Adolescents are swingers, not because they have such active social lives (although they may), but because their behavior and moods may swing so extremely, from the childish dependence of years gone by to the mature independence of adult years approaching. Adolescents are frequently insecure and unstable. The adolescent years tend to be sensitive ones. Resentment and rebellion may arise when needs or desires are thwarted. Closeness is also possible on those occasions when adult understanding is shown. The adolescent usually works hard to become more independent, and asserts his or her independence in front of parents. Adolescents want to be on their own. They want to be able to stand up for themselves. At the same time, they don't want to be too different. Lupus and its treatment can, in many cases, make them feel very different. This can create problems.

For young children, the restrictions of both lupus and its treatment may be unpleasant but tolerable. However, for adolescents living in their "glory days," the changes that accompany lupus may be much more upsetting. Having to experience ongoing pain and to restrict activities, in addition to feeling lethargic and unattractive, may be very depressing for the adolescent.

PERIODS OF REBELLION

Finding out that an adolescent has lupus can cause major problems. The natural tendency of any parent is to become overprotective when a child is sick. Adolescents almost always object to interference from parents. Why? Because the adolescent wants to become more independent. The fact that parents frequently have difficulty dealing with any serious medical condition in their adolescent will, in all likelihood, increase adolescent rebellion. Rebellion is a normal part of adolescence, regardless of whether or not lupus is involved. Parents should try not to be overprotective, but as tolerant and understanding as possible. In cases where the adolescent does something wrong, supportive discussions are more appropriate than put-downs and reproaches.

Rebellion may occasionally lead to more serious physical problems for the adolescent. Why? Because a rebellious teenager may be less diligent with lupus self-care. On occasion, the adolescent may deliberately try to make himself or herself worse, perhaps by not taking the proper medication, by staying out in the sun, or by doing too much (or too little). The adolescent knows that these behaviors can be harmful. Hopefully, he or she will learn (without dangerous consequences) that there are better ways to get through adolescence!

PROBLEMS WITH FRIENDS

Lupus may result in loss of friendships. This can be a problem for anyone, but especially for the adolescent. Making friends is probably one of the most important activities during the adolescent years. Restrictions because of lupus reduce available activities. The adolescent may not be able to spend as much time as desired with friends. It may not be possible to go out as often or keep late hours. It may be necessary to cancel plans at the last minute due to illness. The adolescent may have a hard time deciding whether to tell friends about the illness, and if so, which ones to tell. There may be concern that this information will hurt friendships, new or old. Parents need to be aware of this, so they can try to help. In rare cases, the adolescent might even want teachers to provide short classroom lessons about lupus— what it is and what it can do (after learning themselves, of course!). Hopefully, this will encourage more support and understanding.

EMBARRASSING!

Many adolescents are embarrassed that they have lupus. To an adolescent, any illness can be a stigma. Teenagers have to be O.K. or it may cost them friends (so they believe). What about the stigma of having lupus? Adolescents are at that stage in their lives when social relationships are the most important. They may be less able to get involved in physical activities or go to the gym. They may be more reluctant to develop social relationships because of their concerns about feeling different. All this may create a lot of discomfort in their young minds.

It should, therefore, be up to the adolescent to decide who he or she wants to tell. Teachers should probably know about the illness, since the adolescent may have certain needs or concerns that require more delicate attention. Why might the adolescent choose not to share this information with all friends? He or she might sense that in some cases, friends would be afraid, upset, or even hostile. Some friends might ignore the adolescent, not wanting to be near someone with a chronic medical problem like lupus for fear they might "catch" it. So let your adolescent make the decision.

If the adolescent seems to be having too much difficulty coping with lupus, professional counseling may be helpful. Sometimes, an objective and supportive person can quickly get a troubled adolescent to learn how to adjust to an otherwise emotionally painful disease.

WHO HANDLES IT BETTER?

Many adolescents with lupus cope better than their parents do! Parents may feel guilty. They may feel that they could have done something to prevent their child from having lupus. Parents frequently feel that it is their responsibility to protect their child from harm, disease, or injury. Remember: Adolescents can handle pain more effectively than other age groups, and also deal well with fatigue by resting or pushing themselves in spite of it. The adolescent who feels only some occasional pain and fatigue can usually maintain a fairly normal, active life, despite lupus.

Occasionally, an adolescent may act differently with friends (and in school) than with parents or other family members. Could it be that the adolescent enjoys the protection and concern of parents? The adolescent may put on a different "face" with family than with friends. Isn't that frequently the case, even if lupus isn't involved? Adolescents may be more willing to confide in their parents than in friends. They don't want friends to think they complain all the time.

Some parents try to protect their adolescents by not telling them everything about their conditions. This is usually not the best approach. Adolescents should know the truth, so they can take respon-sibility for their own management. Adjusting to lupus may take a while. By restricting information, parents may hinder their child's adjustment even more. Anger and bitterness between adolescents and their parents may seriously hurt the relationship.

QUESTIONING THE FUTURE

As the adolescent gets older, certain troublesome questions may come to mind. The adolescent may wonder, "Will I be able to marry?" "Will I be able to have children?" "Will I be able to perform my job well enough to keep it?" "Will I be able to make and keep friends?" "Will I be able to finish my education?" "Will I be able to function as a normal member of society?" These questions bother al-most all adolescents. Having lupus just makes them more worrisome. What are the answers? As long as the new condition is taken into con-sideration and the necessary lifestyle changes are made, the adoles-cent with lupus should be just as able to answer these questions as any other healthy teenager.

On to the Future

Well, you've just about finished this book. We've covered a lot of information about lupus. Tremendous progress has been made in treatment for lupus. Earlier diagnosis has led to earlier, more effective treatment, resulting in a better prognosis. Ongoing research continues to test new drugs and techniques for treating the illness, as well as to further improve the quality of life for the person with lupus.

Perhaps by the time you read this, some drug or treatment may have proven itself to be more successful than ones currently available. It remains to be seen which new developments can improve your life with lupus. But at least people are working on the problem. It's nice to know that research continues to investigate ways of improving the effectiveness of treatment.

Although it would be impossible to include every possible problem that might be caused by lupus in this book, I hope that what you've read will help you to develop your own strategies for coping. Because things change and something that troubles you one day may not trouble you the next (and vice versa), you can use this book as a resource. Whenever you have questions about how to cope with a certain aspect of lupus, consult these pages. If you have any comments—information you feel is important—or additional questions, feel free to write to me in care of the publisher. I'd be happy to hear from you.

I hope that within the near future, research will discover a cure for lupus. Then, this book, along with any other book or article written on the subject, could happily be thrown into the fireplace. I look forward to a day when it is no longer needed because lupus no longer exists.

But for now, look brightly ahead, act proudly, and enjoy life as best you can. I wish all of my readers the very best of health and happiness!

Appendix

For Further Reading

Aladjem, H. *Understanding Lupus*. New York: Charles Scribner's Sons, 1985.

Aladjem, H., and Schur, P. *In Search of the Sun*. New York: Charles Scribner's Sons, 1988.

Carr, R. *Lupus Erythematosus: A Handbook for Physicians, Patients, and Their Families*. Washington, DC: Lupus Foundation of America, 1986.

Greater Atlanta Chapter of Lupus Erythematosus Foundation of America. *Lupus Erythematosus*. 4 volumes. Atlanta: Greater Atlanta Chapter of Lupus Erythematosus Foundation of America, 1980, 1981, 1982, 1984.

Lazarus, A. *In the Mind's Eye*. New York: Rawson Associates Publishers, 1977.

For Further Information

Lupus Foundation of America
1717 Massachusetts Avenue, NW
Suite 203
Washington, DC 20036

(800)558-0121

American Lupus Society
23751 Madison Street
Torrance, CA 90505

(213)373-1335

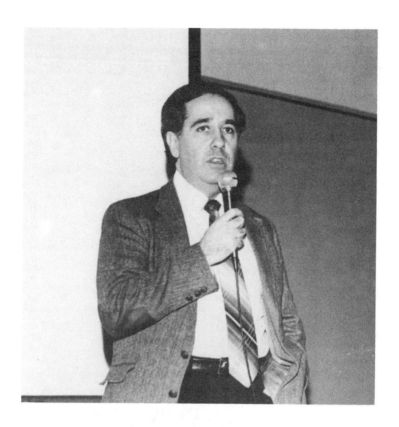

About the Author

Robert H. Phillips, Ph.D., is a practicing psychologist on Long Island, New York. He is the founder and director of the Center for Coping with Chronic Conditions, a multi-service organization helping individuals with chronic illness and their families. In addition, he is the psychologist for and director of the "Cope" program for the Long Island/Queens chapter of the Lupus Foundation of America.

The author of numerous articles on a variety of subjects in psychology, Dr. Phillips has lectured at conventions, universities, and professional meetings throughout the country.

Index